LEARNING GUIDE & JOURNAL
THIRD EDITION

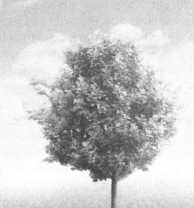

REFLECTIVE PRACTICE

REIMAGINING OURSELVES, REIMAGINING NURSING

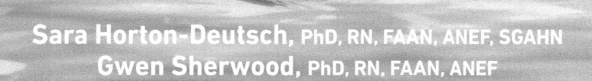

Sara Horton-Deutsch, PhD, RN, FAAN, ANEF, SGAHN
Gwen Sherwood, PhD, RN, FAAN, ANEF

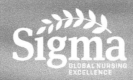

Sigma
GLOBAL NURSING
EXCELLENCE

Sigma Theta Tau International Honor Society of Nursing (Sigma) is a nonprofit organization whose mission is developing nurse leaders anywhere to improve healthcare everywhere. Founded in 1922, Sigma has more than 135,000 active members in over 100 countries and territories. Members include practicing nurses, instructors, researchers, policymakers, entrepreneurs, and others. Sigma's more than 540 chapters are located at more than 700 institutions of higher education throughout Armenia, Australia, Botswana, Brazil, Canada, Chile, Colombia, Croatia, England, Eswatini, Finland, Ghana, Hong Kong, Ireland, Israel, Italy, Jamaica, Japan, Jordan, Kenya, Lebanon, Malawi, Mexico, the Netherlands, Nigeria, Pakistan, Philippines, Portugal, Puerto Rico, Scotland, Singapore, South Africa, South Korea, Sweden, Taiwan, Tanzania, Thailand, the United States, and Wales. Learn more at www.sigmanursing.org.

Sigma Theta Tau International
550 West North Street
Indianapolis, IN, USA 46202

To request a review copy for course adoption, order additional books, buy in bulk, or purchase for corporate use, contact Sigma Marketplace at 888.654.4968 (US/Canada toll-free), +1.317.687.2256 (International), or solutions@sigmamarketplace.org.

To request author information, or for speaker or other media requests, contact Sigma Marketing at 888.634.7575 (US/Canada toll-free) or +1.317.634.8171 (International).

ISBN: 9781646481507
EPUB ISBN: 9781646481514
PDF ISBN: 9781646481521
MOBI ISBN: 9781646481538

Publisher: Dustin Sullivan
Acquisitions Editor: Emily Hatch
Development Editor: Jillmarie Leeper Sycamore
Cover Designer: Rebecca Batchelor
Interior Design/Page Layout: Rebecca Batchelor

Managing Editor: Carla Hall
Publications Specialist: Todd Lothery
Project Editor: Todd Lothery
Copy Editor: Jane Palmer
Proofreader: Todd Lothery

DEDICATION

The *Reflective Practice Learning Guide & Journal* is dedicated to all nurses around the globe who provide selfless care in improving healthcare everywhere.

ACKNOWLEDGMENTS

We acknowledge the partnership and collaboration with the publishing team at Sigma Theta Tau International for their guidance and shared vision in producing this work. We also acknowledge those who have mentored, coached, and educated us towards wholeness and well-being through reflective practices grounded in Caring Science so that nurses everywhere practice to their fullest extent.

ABOUT THE AUTHORS

SARA HORTON-DEUTSCH, PhD, RN, FAAN, ANEF, SGAHN, is a Caritas Coach & Leader, Professor, and Director of the University of San Francisco/Kaiser Permanente Partnership at the University of San Francisco School of Nursing and Health Professions. In this role she coordinates an RN-MSN specialty track for nurse leaders working at one of the 21 Kaiser Permanente hospitals in the Bay Area and collaborates with the Kaiser Permanente Scholars Academy to ensure relevant and quality continuing education programming grounded in Unitary Caring Science. She is also a Faculty Associate at the Watson Caring Science Institute, where she serves as the Co-Director of the Caritas Leadership Program, designed to engage participants in deep study and personal mastery of Caritas leadership, guided by Watson's Caring Science literacy and the 10 Caritas Processes.

Her work in reflective practice has been published in three co-edited books with Gwen Sherwood: *Reflective Practice: Transforming Education and Improving Outcomes* (2012 & 2017) and *Reflective Organizations: On the Front Lines of QSEN and Reflective Practice Implementation* (2015). The second was recognized as an AJN Book of the Year. Clinical nurses and academic programs around the world use the scholarly contributions found in these books to support deep learning—learning that leads to intentional, effective, and thoughtful action. It was through the iterative process of reflection that Horton-Deutsch deepened her own work in reflective practice, resulting in the integration of Caring Science. Like reflective practice, Caring Science calls healthcare professions to action—sacred actions that honor all living things—to health, healing, and wholeness.

In 2022 she co-edited *Visionary Leadership in Healthcare: Excellence in Practice, Policy, and Ethics* with Holly Wei, which received a first-place AJN Book of the Year Award. The textbook is directed toward those who believe centering care and compassion as the foundation for leadership is a worthy endeavor. It invites readers to explore leadership from a holistic perspective, including the knowledge and skills needed but also the social and emotional literacy required. It guides readers on how to be more self-aware, present, engaged, and connected with others to co-create new ways of being and doing our work together.

She continues to influence the scholarship and teaching-learning mindset of nurse educators around the world through her scholarly publications; international, national, and regional presentations; leadership in Caring Science; and service to the profession. She has served as a Research Fellow at the University of South Africa since 2016. In 2022, she was recognized as a Scholar in the Global Academy of Holistic Nursing. Horton-Deutsch currently serves on the board of directors of Sigma.

GWEN D. SHERWOOD, PhD, RN, FAAN, ANEF, has a distinguished record in advancing nursing education locally and globally. She is Professor Emeritus at the University of North Carolina (UNC) at Chapel Hill School of Nursing. She is an expert in patient safety, teamwork, and interprofessional education, and her work focuses on transforming healthcare environments by expanding the relational capacity of healthcare providers. Her work has examined patient satisfaction with pain management outcomes, the spiritual dimensions of care, and teamwork as a variable in patient safety spanning education and practice.

Sherwood was a pioneer in integrating quality and safety in health professions education. She was co-investigator for the award-winning Quality and Safety Education for Nurses (QSEN) project to transform education and practice to prepare nurses to work in and lead quality and safety in redesigned healthcare systems. Funded by the Robert Wood Johnson Foundation from 2005–2012, the QSEN Steering Team received the Sigma Theta Tau International (Sigma) Nursing Media Award, and its website (www.QSEN. org) received the Information Technology Award.

Sherwood has been engaged in multiple interprofessional projects including co-investigator for the UNC-Chapel Hill and Duke University Interprofessional Patient Safety Education Collaborative, patient safety leader at the University of Illinois at Chicago School of Medicine and the Academy for Emerging Leaders in Patient Safety (formerly the Telluride Project), and adjunct faculty in the Master of Science in Patient Safety Leadership program and now the MedStar Patient Safety Institute.

Her professional service includes the Research Committee of the National Patient Safety Foundation, the Technical Expert Panel of TeamSTEPPS, the QSEN Advisory Board, Past President of the International Association for Human Caring, faculty and mentor in the Sigma Nurse Faculty Leadership Academy, and advisor for the Technical Expert Panel for the Patient Centered Care AHRQ Task Order at MedStar Health.

Sherwood's distinguished service to Sigma includes Distinguished Lecturer, Virginia Henderson Fellow, Chair of the global task force for the Scholarship of Reflective Practice position paper, and Vice President of the board of directors. She chaired the Research Scholarship Advisory Council and speaks frequently for chapters around the world. Her hospital research team received the 2001 Regional Research Utilization Award for implementing relationship-centered care.

Her work bridges US and global organizations to expand nursing undergraduate and graduate education capacity to serve developing regions. Formerly Executive Associate Dean at the University of Texas Health Science Center at Houston's School of Nursing, she bridged academia and practice through a joint appointment as Co-Director of the Center for Professional Excellence at The Methodist Hospital. She led numerous educational outreach programs in developing areas both on the Texas-Mexico border and around the world. A global ambassador for nursing, she has worked with nurse educators in Kazakhstan, Sakhalin, Macau, Thailand, Taiwan, and Kenya and helped lead the nursing education renaissance in China.

Widely published, she is co-editor of three other books: *International Textbook of Reflective Practice in Nursing*, *Quality and Safety in Nursing: A Competency Approach to Improve Outcomes* (AJN Book of the Year), and *Reflective Organizations: On the Front Lines of QSEN and Reflective Practice Implementation* (second place AJN Book of the Year). Among many honors, she was awarded Outstanding Alumnus at Georgia Baptist College of Nursing and the University of Texas Austin in addition to the Special Award for International Interprofessional Education from the Prince Madhidol Conference, Sigma's Mary Tolle Wright Leadership Award, an honorary doctorate from Jonkoping University, and Fellowship Ad Eundem from the Royal College of Surgeons Ireland.

CONTRIBUTING AUTHORS

JENNIFER ALDERMAN, PhD, MSN, RN, CNL, CNE, CHSE, is an Associate Professor at the University of North Carolina-Chapel Hill School of Nursing. She holds administrative roles in the undergraduate program and as the School of Nursing's Director of Interprofessional Education and Practice. Alderman's areas of expertise include simulation, interprofessional education, leadership, quality and safety, and maternal/newborn nursing. Alderman has presented nationally and internationally on reflective practice and its role in leadership and transition to practice for new graduate nurses.

GAIL ARMSTRONG, PhD, DNP, RN, ACNS-BC, CNE, FAAN, has been in nursing higher education for more than 20 years. Armstrong has enjoyed a long-standing interest in reflective practice as her first two degrees are in literature. Early in her career, she was a med/surg bedside nurse where an interest in illness narratives united her work as a nurse and her foundation in Caring Science. Much of Armstrong's career focused on quality and safety and the integration of quality and safety content into early pre-licensure curricula. Armstrong found reflective practice to be fertile pedagogy for pre-licensure students to reflect on and respond to system gaps they were observing in their clinical rotations. In her current work as Faculty Development Coordinator, Armstrong supports the growth and development of CU Nursing faculty in all phases of their careers.

ANNA BILEY, Dip N, MSc, Doctorate of Caring Science, has worked across a range of specialties in clinical, leadership, and educational roles in the UK's National Health Service and in the voluntary sector. At the heart of her work has been understanding and developing Watson Caring Science and Human Caring Theory. Recent years brought personal change and challenge as Biley became a full-time mum and carer for close family members. During this time, she undertook the doctoral program at the Watson Caring Science Institute (WCSI) and as faculty now supports the Caritas Coach and Leadership programs. Grief, loss, and recovery are the focus of her most recent work and writing. A book based on her doctoral research, entitled *Birds Hold our Secrets: A Nurse's Story of Grief and Remembering,* was published in 2019 by Lotus Library (WCSI).

DAWN FRESHWATER, PhD, RN, FRCN, FRCSI, MAE, GAICD, is Vice-Chancellor of the University of Auckland. She was the first female Chair of the G08 Research Intensive Universities in Australia and the past Chair of the Partnership Board of the World University Network (WUN). Freshwater is currently Chair of UNZ Research Committee and Deputy Chair and Board Director of Research Australia. She was awarded her PhD at the University of Nottingham (1998). Her contribution to the fields of nursing, public health (specifically mental health and forensic mental health), and research on leadership practices won her the highest honor in her field—the Fellowship of the Royal College of Nursing (FRCN). Freshwater is an elected Member of the Academia Europea and a Fellow of the Royal College of Surgeons Ireland. As an academic, she has contributed to more than 200 publications, including peer-reviewed papers, research reports, books, editorials, and media contributions, and she continues to supervise PhD students. Freshwater maintains strong professional ties with key figures in education and industry in Asia, Europe, and the United States. She is known for her advocacy and action for equity and inclusivity.

EILEEN FRY-BOWERS, PhD, JD, RN, CPNP-PC, FAAN, is Dean and Professor at the University of San Francisco School of Nursing and Health Professions. Her academic experience includes faculty and leadership appointments in Schools of Nursing, Medicine, and Public Health, and her extensive clinical experience spans multiple healthcare settings, including acute care facilities, specialty and community-based clinics, and military institutions. She is a certified pediatric nurse practitioner (CPNP), a licensed attorney, and a veteran of the US Navy Nurse Corps. Fry-Bowers is an elected Fellow of the American Academy of Nursing and former Chair of the Expert Panel on Child, Adolescent, and Family. She was named a Faculty Policy Fellow for the American Association of Colleges of Nursing and served two terms on AACN's Health Policy Advisory Council. Fry-Bowers is committed to transforming nursing education and practice to support the promotion, development, and maintenance of optimal mental, physical, and spiritual health for all, including the nursing workforce.

CHRISTINE GRIFFIN, PhD, RN, NPD-BC, CPN, is the Director of Caring Science and Nursing Practice at Queens Medical Center in Honolulu, Hawaii. In her PhD program, "Compassion Without Fatigue," Griffin studied how the theory-guided practices within Caring Science can inform effective compassion fatigue interventions to decrease burnout for healthcare providers. As faculty for the Watson Caring Science Institute and a Caritas Coach and leader, she hopes to bring Caring Science practices to nurses and nurse leaders so they have the capacity to flourish as they bring their authentic care and compassion to the bedside. Griffin has contributed to Caring Science and leadership chapters in *Caritas Coaching: A Journey Toward Transpersonal Caring for Informed Moral Action in Healthcare* (2018), *Nursing Theories and Nursing Practice,* 5th Edition (2020), and *Leadership Roles in Promoting a Resilient Workforce* (2022).

CAROLE HEMMELGARN, MS, is the Director of the Executive Master's program for Clinical Quality, Safety & Leadership at Georgetown University and the Senior Director of Education for the MedStar Health Institute for Quality & Safety. Hemmelgarn graduated from Colorado State University with a degree in Speech Communication. She received a master's degree in Patient Safety Leadership from the University of Illinois at Chicago and a second master's degree in Health Care Ethics from Creighton University. Hemmelgarn is involved in patient safety work across the country. She sits on the Leapfrog Patient & Family Caregiver Expert Panel; the Board of Quality, Safety, and Experience at Children's Hospital Colorado; the Clinical Excellence Council for Colorado Hospital Association; ABIM Foundation; the Patient Advisory Committee and the board of directors for the Collaborative for Accountability and Improvement; and is a founding member of Patients For Patient Safety US.

ERICA HOOPER, DNP, RN, CNL,CNS, PHN, is a Regional Program Manager for Academic Relations and Community Health for the Kaiser Permanente Scholars Academy in Northern California and adjunct faculty at the University of San Francisco School of Nursing and Health Professions. She has nursing experience working in the areas of geriatrics, pediatrics, primary care, public health, leadership, program development, and education. She has a BSN and DNP in Health Care Systems Leadership from the University of San Francisco and an MSN in Advanced Community Health and International Nursing with a minor in Education from the University of California San Francisco. Hooper is a Caritas Coach, HeartMath certified trainer, healing circle facilitator, massage and reiki practitioner, yoga instructor, personal trainer, and life coach. She has a passion for alternative healing practices as well as promoting the health and wellness of vulnerable populations. Hooper has a personal mission in life to use her gifts to help others achieve their greatest potential and healthiest version of themselves.

ASHLEY A. KELLISH, DNP, RN, CCNS, NEA-BC, is an academic and clinical practitioner dedicated to the future of nurses in healthcare. Her experience has allowed her to provide mentorship to over 20 DNP and MSN candidates through the University of North Carolina (UNC) Medical School of Chapel Hill, North Carolina. She is a sought-after consultant with a propensity for implementing change and improving healthcare systems. She has formally presented and led workshops throughout the United States and globally on continuing education and shifting protocols. Kellish earned her DNP from Duke University, an MSN from Georgetown University, where she was awarded Performance Improvement Nurse of the Year, and a bachelor's degree in nursing from Boston College. She is a board-certified Critical Care Clinical Nurse Specialist. In 2022, she was honored by UNC as a member of the third cohort of Anne Belcher Interprofessional Faculty Scholars. She also holds many certifications and has authored publications on nursing, systems, and practices.

JENNIFER MANEY, PhD, is the Director of the Center for Teaching and Learning at Marquette University. Her role is to support all faculty/instructors in promoting a welcoming learning environment through their pedagogical practices, including the infusion of Ignatian principles into their teaching. She is responsible for helping to build inclusive, equitable, and justice-focused learning experiences across campus, and facilitating faculty exploration of the impact of implicit biases. Maney currently teaches in the first-year honors program at Marquette University, is adjunct faculty for Mount Mary College, and is the board chair of St. Joan Antida Catholic High School. Prior, she was responsible for the coordination of the Greater Milwaukee Catholic Education Consortium in support of Milwaukee K-12 Catholic schools. She has experience directing a federal grant at the Milwaukee Area Technical College, helping to create the first bilingual early childhood credential program in the state of Wisconsin. She holds a doctorate in Educational Policy and Leadership with a minor in diversity education, a master's in counseling, and a bachelor's degree in journalism.

MEG MOORMAN, PhD, RN, CNE, ANEF, is the Coordinator of the MSN in Nursing Education Program and the Director of the Faculty Innovating for Nursing Education (FINE) Research Center at Indiana University School of Nursing. Prior to teaching, she worked as a labor and delivery nurse and nurse practitioner. Her research has focused on interactive teaching strategies, mostly focused on Visual Thinking Strategies (VTS) and the use of art to teach communication, observational skills, ethics, and diversity. Moorman has been the recipient of several teaching awards including the IU Trustees Teaching Award, Sigma Theta Tau Excellence in Nursing Education (Alpha Chapter) Award, and the Mosaic Teaching Fellowship. She has presented and consulted internationally with schools of nursing, medicine, education, and palliative care groups. Her research has been disseminated in Hong Kong, South Africa, Spain, Ireland, and Australia, and she has worked with several hospital systems to introduce VTS into nurse residency programs.

CRYSTAL MORALES, MS, BSN, RN, is the Director of Nurse Wellbeing at MedStar Health. Dedicated to nurses' well-being, she has the privilege of developing and implementing strategies aimed at improving professional, emotional, physical, and social well-being. Morales has a strong and extensive background in healthcare management, operations, and education. Most recently she served as the Senior Director of Education at the MedStar Institute for Quality and Safety. In that role, she was the acting Program Director for Georgetown's Executive Master's in Clinical Quality, Safety, and Leadership program. Prior to that, Morales held various roles at MedStar, where she skillfully led the development and implementation of system-wide strategies for high reliability and patient safety. Morales is exceptionally passionate about her work and enjoys making connections and working on diverse teams.

DANIEL J. PESUT, PhD, RN, FAAN, is a nurse educator, academic, researcher, consultant, and coach. He is an Emeritus Professor of Nursing at the University of Minnesota School of Nursing and Emeritus Katherine R. and C. Walton Lillehei Chair in Nursing Leadership at the University of Minnesota. He has held academic and administrative positions at the University of Michigan, the University of South Carolina, and Indiana University. He served as the Director of the Katharine J. Densford International Center for Nursing Leadership from 2012 until his retirement in 2021. He is a past President (2003–2005) of Sigma Theta Tau International. His Presidential Call to Action was "Create the Future Through Renewal." The Sigma Daniel J. Pesut Spirit of Renewal Award honors his leadership and legacy contributions to the nursing profession.

MELISSA SHEW, PhD, is a Senior Faculty Fellow in Marquette University's Center for Teaching and Learning, Faculty Director of the Executive MBA Program, and Co-Director of Marquette's Institute for Women and Leadership. She works in the history of philosophy, feminist philosophy, philosophy of education, and issues related to women at work. Her recent scholarship includes *Philosophy for Girls: An Invitation to the Life of Thought* (with Kim Garchar, Oxford University Press, 2020); *On the Vocation of the Educator in This Moment* (with Jennifer Maney, Marquette University Press, 2021); a TEDx Talk, "Women and Intellectual Empowerment" (2021); a white paper, "The Power of Intellectual Joy for the Future of Women at Work" (2023); and a creative public-facing research initiative, *The Persephone Project* (https://thepersephoneproject.org/).

GISELA H. VAN RENSBURG, DLitt et Phil, RN, RM, RPN, RCN, RNE, RNA, ROrthN, FANSA, obtained her DLitt et Phil at the University of South Africa, where she is a Professor in the Department of Health Studies. She serves as the Master's and Doctoral Program Coordinator and member of the Human Sciences Research Ethics Committee. She holds a grant for a Women in a Research project on psycho-educational support strategies for postgraduate supervisors and students to facilitate mental well-being. van Rensburg has engaged in a variety of research projects on research capacity development and teaching research methodology. She is an editor of two research books. Her current international research partnership involves reflective practices and Caring Science related to teaching and learning. As an educator, van Rensburg focuses on health sciences education, student support, and reflective practice. Her clinical interests are in orthopaedic nursing, in which she holds a specialist nursing qualification. She mentors members of the nursing community in research capacity development, with a special interest in supporting novices and emerging researchers.

ROBIN R. WALTER, PhD, RN, CNE, is contributing faculty in the DNP and PhD nursing programs at Walden University. She is a nurse educator with experience in health and public policy, committed to developing nurses as leaders in equity policy advocacy and as social justice allies. Her research on health disparities and inequities is anchored in understanding the political determinants of health that create inequities in the social determinants of health. Walter has developed curricula and courses conceptually grounded in social justice, diversity, equity, and inclusion at the baccalaureate, master's, and doctoral levels of nursing education. She co-led a grant-funded initiative in Florida to prepare nurse leaders across the state to engage in equity policy advocacy. Walter earned a BSN from Towson University, an MS in nursing/health policy from the University of Maryland at Baltimore, and a PhD in nursing from Barry University.

AMBER YOUNG-BRICE, PhD, RN, CNE, is an Assistant Professor in Nursing and Program Director of the Teaching Certificate for Nurse Educators program at Marquette University. She holds a master's degree in nursing education, PhD in nursing, and is a certified nurse educator. She has taught at the undergraduate, graduate, and post-graduate levels since 2008. Additionally, Young-Brice does educational development across the university and within her college of nursing as a new faculty mentor and conducts programming for onboarding all new faculty. Young-Brice's program of pedagogical research explores the relationship between the influence of non-cognitive factors and the successful trajectory of students. She studies ways to foster these factors through theoretically derived and evidence-informed pedagogical innovations. Her research is grounded in her expertise as an educator and underpinned by theories from nursing, education, and cognitive and social sciences. She is the 2018 NLN Ruth Donnelly Corcoran Research Award recipient and principal investigator on a 2023 NSF-funded study integrating human-centered teaching practices in engineering education.

SPECIAL NOTE TO READERS

Here at Sigma, we realize that language is constantly evolving. The meaning of a word often changes over time, some words become obsolete, and some terms that were once acceptable may become controversial or even offensive, depending on the context or circumstances. We have made every effort to make language choices that are inclusive and not offensive. Should you identify words in this book that you believe negatively impact a group or groups of people, please reach out to us at Publications@SigmaNursing.org.

TABLE OF CONTENTS

About the Authors...v

Contributing Authors...vii

Special Note to Readers...xiii

How to Use This Guide..xix

1 REIMAGINING OURSELVES: THE ROLE OF REFLECTION ON CRITICAL CARITAS CONSCIOUSNESS AND KNOWLEDGE DEVELOPMENT 1

Before You Begin...2

Microbpractices...3

Learning Narrative..4

Reflective Questions..5

References...6

2 REIMAGINING REFLECTION TO DEVELOP AND SUSTAIN PERSONAL AND PROFESSIONAL PRACTICE 8

Before You Begin...9

Microbpractices...11

Learning Narrative..13

Reflective Questions..14

References...15

3 REIMAGINING CREATIVE SPACE FOR REFLECTION IN A CARING SCIENCE PARADIGM 16

Before You Begin...17

Microbpractices and Learning Activities...17

Learning Narrative..21

Reflective Questions..22

References...23

4 SELF-REFLECTION THROUGH THE LENS OF UNITARY CARING SCIENCE: LEARNING TO LISTEN AND LISTENING TO LEARN 24

Before You Begin...25

Microbpractices and Learning Activities...26

Learning Narrative..27

Reflective Questions..30

References...31

5 DEEPENING OUR FOUNDATIONS: REIMAGINING OURSELVES, REIMAGINING NURSING IDENTITY **32**

    Before You Begin 33

    Micropractices 34

    Learning Narrative 38

    Reflective Questions 39

    References 40

6 THE ROLE OF REFLECTION IN GUIDING THE EVOLUTION OF CARE, COMPASSION, AND SOCIAL CHANGE **41**

    Before You Begin 42

    Micropractices 43

    Learning Narrative 47

    Reflective Questions 48

    References 48

7 SHARING OUR STORIES: CO-CREATING LEARNING THROUGH NARRATIVE PEDAGOGY, SILENCE, AND LISTENING **49**

    Before You Begin 50

    Micropractices 50

    Reflective Questions 55

    References 57

8 REIMAGINING PRACTICING TOGETHER: REFLECTION IN SIMULATION-BASED LEARNING **58**

    Before You Begin 59

    Micropractices 60

    Learning Narrative 62

    Reflective Questions 64

    References 65

9 REFLECTIVE LEARNING: RECALIBRATING COLLABORATION AND EVALUATION FOR SAFETY AND QUALITY COMPETENCIES **66**

    Before You Begin 67

    Micropractices 67

    Learning Narrative 71

    Reflective Questions 73

    References 74

10 RETHINKING HOW WE WORK TOGETHER: REFLECTIVE PRACTICES USING EMERGENT STRATEGY, LIBERATING STRUCTURES, AND CLEARNESS COMMITTEES 75

Before You Begin 76

Micropractices 77

Learning Narrative 79

Reflective Questions...81

References 82

11 PLURALISTIC POSSIBILITY: REFLECTIVE PRACTICES TO REFRAME OUR WORLD. 83

Before You Begin 84

Micropractices 85

Learning Narrative 87

Reflective Questions...88

References 89

12 REDESIGNING ACADEMIC AND PRACTICE PARTNERSHIPS: REFLECTIVE COMMUNITIES THAT LEARN AND PRACTICE TOGETHER 90

Before You Begin 91

Micropractices 91

Learning Narrative 92

Reflective Questions...94

References 95

13 THE VALUE OF EMANCIPATORY NURSING PRAXIS AND CARING SCIENCE IN AN ERA OF LEGISLATIVE CENSORSHIP 96

Before You Begin 97

Micropractices 98

Learning Narrative 100

Reflective Questions... 102

References 104

14 REIMAGINING LEADERSHIP: A LEGACY PERSPECTIVE 105

Before You Begin 106

Micropractices 106

Learning Narrative by Dan Pesut 107

Reflective Questions... 109

References 111

15   REFLECTIVE PRACTICE, UNITARY CARING SCIENCE, AND WISDOM: THE HEART OF THE CAPACITY TO GROW **112**

Before You Begin 113

Micropractices 114

Learning Narrative 118

Reflective Questions... 119

References 120

HOW TO USE THIS GUIDE

This guide is a companion and stand-alone resource for integrating the teachings and learnings from *Reflective Practice: Reimagining Ourselves, Reimagining Nursing*. Reflection is crucial for personal and professional growth and development as it allows us to analyze and learn from our experiences. By reflecting on past events, particularly in light of the pain, suffering, and loss from COVID-19 and our healthcare systems' ongoing inadequacies and inequities, we can identify what went well and works well and what needs improvement. In turn, this knowledge can help us make better future decisions. Reflection also allows us to recognize patterns in our behavior and thought processes, which can be valuable in improving relationships, reconnecting to values and purpose, and taking risks to achieve goals. Therefore, instilling the "habit of the mind" to reflect regularly can significantly influence our sense of purpose, overall well-being, and growth.

The following terms frame the learning embedded in the textbook and this learning guide. This language may be new to some readers but is intentional as we seek a more human-centered and caring literate approach to healthcare grounded in care, compassion, and the theoretical foundations of the nursing discipline.

LEARNING OBJECTIVES/SUBJECTIVES

Each chapter begins with learning objectives and subjectives to emphasize the importance of fully integrating cognitive, psychomotor, and affective learning into our teaching and learning. Studies demonstrate that education does not occur without considering emotions (American Association of Colleges of Nursing, 2021; Immordino-Yang, 2016; Thompson & Carello, 2022). To create optimal learning environments, educators must acknowledge, guide, and role-model ways to manage the emotional context of learning and practice to incorporate the spectrum of clinical and professional experiences into learning activities.

MICROPRACTICES

Definitions of micropractices are not widely established within the nursing academic or professional literature. For the purposes of this learning guide, we define *micropractices* as small-scale practices or actions carried out with specific goals or intentions. Within the textbook and this learning guide, micropractices guide reflective practice activities seeking to achieve deeper insights and understandings in a specific area of care for self or others. Micropractices offer:

- **Accessibility and convenience:** Micropractices are designed to be easily accessible and readily utilized. Learners can access these short activities at their own pace and opportunities, making learning more convenient.

- **Engagement and focus:** The short duration of micropractices helps maintain learner engagement and focus. Learners are less likely to experience cognitive overload as the content is concise and to the point.

- **Retention and reinforcement:** Frequent exposure to key concepts through micropractices aids retention and reinforces learning. Short learning intervals spread over time reinforce learning and enhance long-term memory retention.

- **Flexibility and personalization:** Micropractices enable learners to customize their learning experience based on their interests and needs. Learners can choose micropractices matched with their learning needs, tailoring their learning journey accordingly.

- **Skill development:** Micropractices are effective for skill development, particularly regarding practical or hands-on skills. Short, focused exercises allow learners the opportunity to practice and refine their abilities.

- **Time efficiency:** Traditional learning methods often involve long lectures or training sessions, requiring a significant time commitment. Micropractices deliver content in brief chunks, allowing learners to advance even in short periods so they can continually assess their progress.

- **Continuous and lifelong learning:** Micropractices encourage a culture of continuous learning and support lifelong learning habits. By instilling these short reflective learning activities as a mindful habit, learners practice the professional standard of continuous learning and engagement over the course of their career.

LEARNING NARRATIVE

Using the language associated with *learning narratives* provides distinct advantages over the traditional case study method in certain situations. Learning narratives enrich teaching by providing a more holistic, empathetic, and contextually grounded perspective within the learning process. Key values of using the language of learning narratives include:

- **Contextual understanding:** Learning narratives often focus on the experience of individuals or groups as they navigate the process of learning. This approach allows for a more in-depth exploration of the cultural, social, and emotional factors influencing education. As a result, it provides a richer and more contextual understanding of the learning process compared to a case study that might be more detached and objective.

- **Personal perspective:** The language of learning narratives brings a unique person-centered perspective to the forefront, which can create empathy, compassion, and connection with learners and serves as a foundation for relationship-centered care. These narratives are often told in first-person or through interviews, enabling learners to relate to the challenges, successes, and feelings more directly.

- **Emphasis on process:** While case studies typically focus on analyzing a specific case or situation, learning narratives are learning-oriented. This process-oriented approach assists educators and learners in gaining insights into strategies, obstacles, and development over time.

- **Inspiration and motivation:** Reading or listening to learning narratives can be inspiring for learners. Hearing success stories, overcoming challenges, and seeing the journey of others can instill a sense of determination and dedication in learners, fostering a positive learning environment.

- **Cultural and linguistic diversity:** Learning narratives often encompass diverse languages, cultures, and linguistic backgrounds. By exploring narratives from various perspectives, learners can gain a broader appreciation for diverse cultures, fostering cross-cultural understanding and sensitivity in co-creating person-centered and relationship-centered approaches for learners, self, and peers.

- **Qualitative insights:** Learning narratives offer qualitative or experiential insights that delve into the emotions, thoughts, and experiences of learners that complement the more quantitative and objective nature of case studies. These experiential, human-centered insights complement the data-driven approach of case studies, providing a more comprehensive approach to learning.

REFLECTIVE QUESTIONS

Reflective questions are crucial in knowledge application, encouraging deeper thinking, self-assessment, and critical analysis. They encourage learners to review and evaluate their experiences, knowledge, and skills, leading to more meaningful and sustained learning outcomes. Incorporating reflective questions into the learning process is a powerful tool for enhancing learning outcomes, promoting personal growth, and fostering a deeper understanding of the subject matter. Reflective questions embrace fundamental values for:

- **Promoting critical thinking:** Reflective questions prompt learners to think critically about what they have learned, how it applies to real-life situations, and the reasons behind specific outcomes. This helps them develop a deeper understanding of the subject matter.

- **Encouraging self-awareness:** Reflective questions encourage self-awareness by guiding learners to examine their strengths, weaknesses, and areas for improvement. This introspection can lead to better self-regulation and goal-setting in the learning process.

- **Fostering metacognition:** Reflective questions prompt learners to think about their thinking (metacognition). This metacognitive awareness helps them become more effective learners, as they can identify their learning strategies and adapt them accordingly.

- **Enhancing retention and application:** When learners reflect on what they have learned, they are more likely to retain and transfer the information to new contexts. The act of making connections between new knowledge and existing knowledge solidifies learning.

- **Building problem-solving skills:** By reflecting on challenges and problem-solving approaches, learners can identify alternative solutions and develop a more adaptive and flexible mindset.

- **Encouraging continuous improvement:** Reflective questions continually push learners to improve their knowledge and skills. They identify areas of strength and areas that need work, leading to a growth mindset and a commitment to lifelong learning.

- **Supporting deeper engagement:** Learners who are encouraged to reflect become more engaged with the learning process. This active engagement enhances motivation and the overall learning experience.

- **Promoting empathy and understanding:** Reflective questions can also be applied to interpersonal and social learning. By encouraging learners to reflect on their interactions with others, they can develop empathy, understanding, and better communication skills.

- **Facilitating feedback:** Reflective questions allow learners to seek and receive feedback from educators, mentors, or peers. Constructive feedback can help learners identify blind spots and areas for improvement.

- **Strengthening decision-making skills:** Reflective thinking helps learners make informed decisions by considering various factors, potential consequences, and alternatives.

PUTTING IT INTO PRACTICE

The *Reflective Practice Learning Guide & Journal* can stand alone or serve as an accompaniment to the full textbook, *Reflective Practice: Reimagining Ourselves, Reimagining Nursing,* Third Edition. Whether you are a learner, an educator, or a nurse, this guide provides the tools and strategies as micropractices for deepening your understanding of what it is to be a nurse, develop self-awareness in emotional intelligence, and attune to personal knowing to inform your moral, ontological, and intellectual capacities in whatever way you practice nursing. Across the professional nurse continuum, everyone needs a mindset of intentionally responding to and balancing the professional challenges in building a strong foundation and source of renewal. Learners may use the book as part of a class, as a personal approach to renewal and revisioning, or as a part of systematic professional growth and development. Educators can use the guide for their own professional development, renewal, and regeneration or as an accompaniment to classroom or clinical learning experiences with any level of learner. Both learners and educators can lead journal clubs, interest groups, or study groups using this learning guide and journal. Wherever you are in nursing, this book is a way forward into reimagining yourself and reimagining nursing to cultivate a critical awareness of who you are, what values you live, and the attitudes that guide the choices you make.

Teaching and practicing nursing are relational endeavors; thus, relationships play a crucial role in understanding the complexity of nursing practice and the way we work together inter- and intra-professionally. Engage in this reflective practice guide to find your voice, create environments fostering belonging and equity, experience satisfaction, and model care science in your work every day, wherever that may be.

REFERENCES

American Association of Colleges of Nursing. (2021). *The essentials: Core competencies for professional nursing education.* https://www.aacnnursing.org/Portals/42/AcademicNursing/pdf/Essentials-2021.pdf

Immordino-Yang, M. H. (2016). *Ed-Talk: Learning with an emotional brain* [Video]. YouTube. American Educational Research Association. https://www.youtube.com/watch?v=DEeo350WQrs

Thompson, P., & Carello, J. (2022). *Trauma-informed pedagogies: A guide for responding to crisis and inequality in healthcare.* Palgrave Macmillan.

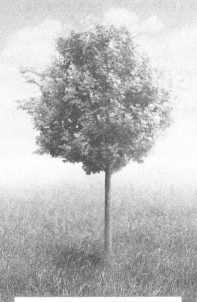

CHAPTER 1

REIMAGINING OURSELVES: THE ROLE OF REFLECTION ON CRITICAL CARITAS CONSCIOUSNESS AND KNOWLEDGE DEVELOPMENT

Dawn Freshwater, PhD, RN, FRCN, FRCSI, MAE, GAICD
Sara Horton-Deutsch, PhD, RN, FAAN, ANEF, SGAHN
Gwen Sherwood, PhD, RN, FAAN, ANEF

LEARNING OBJECTIVES/SUBJECTIVES

- Identify converging societal and technological issues impacting knowledge development.

- Explore theoretical frameworks that guide reflection, critical Caritas consciousness, and Caritas literacy.

- Explain the role of reflection, critical Caritas consciousness, and Caritas literacy in addressing complex issues in nursing.

- Appraise the value of relational learning for the development of more socially and culturally conscious and morally courageous nurses.

BEFORE YOU BEGIN

Reflective Practice: Reimagining Ourselves, Reimagining Nursing, Third Edition, arose in the aftermath of social, cultural, professional, and educational disruption experienced in the COVID-19 pandemic. Change and disruption from emerging technology, social justice issues, and educational shifts were simply accelerated into an avalanche overwhelming nurses, educators, learners, and the population at large. The book is a road map for each of us as we grapple with emerging paradigms that are unfamiliar, yet we are compelled towards adaptation to continue to meet the goals of education and practice.

Part I explores the development, evolution, and imperative for integrating reflective practices into nursing education and healthcare. Reflective practices provide lifelong learning tools to engage nurses in building a strong foundation for their work and intentionally instill habits of renewal and regeneration.

Chapter 1 dissects the converging societal and technological issues impacting knowledge development to guide educators, nurses, and learners in responding to paradigm shifts in teaching and curriculum, healthcare delivery systems, and professional practice models. To prepare for these transitions, each of us is encouraged to explore multiple perspectives through transformative learning experiences that integrate reflective practices that expand self-awareness and motivate changes in behavior.

The chapter explains theoretical underpinning including critical literacy (Watson, 2017), emancipatory learning (Friere, 2000), transformative learning (Mezirow & Taylor, 2009; Van Schalkwyk et al., 2019), and Unitary Caring Science and relational learning (Watson, 2018). Lee (2017) states that Caritas literacy guides development of skills such as centering, authentic presence, deep listening, reflection, and deeper consciousness—thus, the antidote to nurse burnout.

Unitary Caring Science provides the lens through which educators, nurses, and learners deepen reflection in and on practice, balance "doing" with "being" in promoting a relational way of working together, and develop productive approaches for managing complexity and uncertainty (Watson, 2018). The 10 Caritas Processes are pivotal in developing caring consciousness for balancing exploding technology and artificial intelligence (Wallace et al., 2022) to maintain humanity in nursing and healthcare. Nurses face constant pressures to remain true to moral and ethical practice, calling forth moral courage in striving for right action (International Council of Nursing and Midwifery, 2022; Khodaveisi et al., 2021). Right action is not always comfortable; sometimes it requires courage in the face of potential alienation from peers and colleagues, resulting in stress, anxiety, fear of being scolded, rejection, and seclusion (Khoshmehr et al., 2020). Through critical consciousness, we are faced with questions:

> What constructs your thinking in confronting moral dilemmas in your work? How do you begin to construct sense-making of ethical and moral dilemmas?

> How do you ensure decisions are in the best interest of the patient or learners?

> How do we balance patient safety and quality with the limitations of our own humanity and self-care?

Now is the time for reimagining ourselves by reflecting, learning, and identifying ways to rejuvenate, refresh, revitalize, and reframe our self and our profession. Deepening self-awareness and self-consciousness are part of nurturing interpersonal and intersubjective connections and relations. Nurses enhance their resilience and compassion as caring-healing practitioners by aligning actions with purpose and fulfillment, also known as *praxis*.

The micropractices detailed in this chapter help nurses in applying relational learning, critical theory, and transformative learning guided by the principles and practices of Unitary Caring Science so that their personal and professional lives cultivate a greater sense of self-awareness, relational competence, and agency for navigating complex social and cultural contexts with greater confidence, courage, and resilience. As such, Brindley (2020) argues that in these emerging new paradigms, we have fresh opportunities to reflect on practice through critical caring consciousness, Caritas literacy, and moral courage—together they are the heart of high-quality, evidence-informed nursing care using the development of knowledge situated in a relational ethic.

MICROPRACTICES

FOR INDIVIDUAL REFLECTION AND/OR GROUP DISCUSSION/ JOURNAL CLUB

1. In what ways can the principles of Unitary Caring Science, such as presence, intentionality, and mutual respect, be applied to relational learning in education to foster more holistic and authentic learning experiences for learners?

    _____

    _____

2. How does relational learning inform and guide individual and organizational responses to urgent and complex issues such as food waste, reducing admissions, expanding community care, telehealth, and technology-enhanced learning?

    _____

    _____

3. How can relational learning be used in academic and practice settings to reach and reconcile with marginalized and vulnerable groups, improve access to digital healthcare, and improve culturally appropriate care?

    _____

    _____

4. How can culturally diverse and indigenous knowledge systems inform and help to solve the world's greatest sustainability challenges?

_____

_____

5. How does relational learning in education share similarities with the principles of Unitary Caring Science in healthcare, such as the importance of connection, relationship-building, and compassion in promoting learning and healing?

_____

_____

The following exemplar in the learning narrative details how one educational institution acted with moral courage in developing a relational university-wide curriculum.

LEARNING NARRATIVE

Putting it into practice: Knowledge development through a reflective curriculum model of relational learning.

The University of Auckland's (2022) novel curriculum framework recognizes that excellence in teaching and research is necessary for, and provides a means of, engendering transformation in the lives of many people. Putting the learner at the center of learning and teaching, it recognizes and values their social and emotional selves alongside their academic contributions and through the intersectionality of their often complex lives.

It seeks to create an individual, personalized experience for students in a collective environment, while also supporting staff to innovate purposefully to meet the changing demands of tertiary education and of healthcare settings. The curriculum framework reflects the underpinning principles and approaches highlighted in the university strategy, _Taumata Teitei_, including the role of indigenous knowledge; Te Tiriti o Waitangi principles and accountabilities; Māori pedagogies; research-led and research-informed teaching; sustainability; transdisciplinarity, innovation, and entrepreneurship; and work- and community-integrated learning and practices. It also reflects academic, cultural, social, and emotional strengths and needs within the curriculum; fundamentally, it is built on the foundation of relational learning.

Relational learning (and teaching) refers to practices that invite both learners and educators to enter a dialogue about learning. Key aspects include relationships, interactivity, interactions, connections, communication, and learners' interests. Relational learning recognizes the differences—across culture, gender, physicality, and neurodiversity—as strengths in understanding knowledge from diverse, situated perspectives.

Importantly, relational learning demands an education model that goes beyond the transmission of information, requiring learners to take an active role in the learning process, and encompasses a range of different practices. There is no necessary binary between online and in-person learning in terms of delivering relational learning.

Relational learning is also aligned with *technology-enhanced learning* (TEL), used to describe the application of technology to teaching and learning activities, signaling the value that technology adds to learning in both practice settings and the formal learning environment. TEL is an umbrella term covering all types of teaching and learning delivery, including blended, flexible, multimodal, online, and face-to-face learning. It can foster rich online and in-person experiences and open new avenues for learning, and it helps educate nurses and professionals for the present while empowering them for lifelong learning.

Like many institutions of higher education, the University of Auckland has an aspiration for learners to make the world better tomorrow than it is today. To this end, the university's graduate profile articulates students' educational journey toward this goal through several themes. One theme, *Waipapa ki Uta: The Landing Place,* is highly relevant to sustainability ambitions, speaking as it does to connecting to place for sustainable and enduring partnerships and fostering a range of related capabilities.

With a curriculum that is underpinned by principles of cultural identity, social justice, ecological awareness, and civic duty and which demonstrates sustainable practices and positive outcomes for our communities, we foster graduates who are interculturally aware and connected to their local and global communities. This has essential benefits for our health professionals and for nurses, who practice culturally competent care in one of the most diverse cities in the world.

Many hospital settings and public health environs now have carbon zero and sustainability strategies, some focused on energy and many focused on food waste, reducing admissions, pushing back to community care, and telehealth, with TEL being critical to nurse education and also to preparing nurses for new ways of working as they will develop the skills of helping patients to access increasingly digital healthcare services.

REFLECTIVE QUESTIONS

1. In what ways has the COVID-19 pandemic highlighted the necessity for transformative and relational learning in academic and practice settings?

   _____

   _____

2. Why are ontological competencies (Caritas literacies) vital to the future of nursing and other healthcare professions?

   _____

   _____

3. What new insights have emerged through nurses' relationships with patients and colleagues during the pandemic, and how can these insights inform future approaches to nursing practice and education?

_____

_____

4. How can nurses use the principles of Caring Science to shape their personal/professional development and growth in response to the pandemic, and in doing so, enhance their sense of self-awareness and strengthen relationships with others?

_____

_____

5. What are examples of moral courage you have demonstrated or have observed in advocating for patients and their families during the pandemic, particularly in situations where patients' rights and dignity were at risk?

_____

_____

6. How can nurses foster a culture of moral courage and ethical decision-making within their healthcare teams, and what strategies can they use to encourage others to speak up and take action in the face of ethical challenges?

_____

_____

REFERENCES

Brindley, J. (2020). Reflecting on nursing practice during the COVID-19 pandemic. _Nursing Standard_. https://doi.org/10.7748/ns.2020.e11569

Freire, P. (2000). _Pedagogy of the oppressed_. The Continuum Publishing Company.

International Council of Nurses. (2021). _The ICN code of ethics for nurses_. https://www.icn.ch/system/files/2021-10/ICN_Code-of-Ethics_EN_Web_0.pdf

Khodaveisi, M., Oshvandi, K., Bashirian, S., Khazaei, S., Gillespie, M., Masoumi, S. Z., & Mohammadi, F. (2021). Moral courage, moral sensitivity and safe nursing care in nurses caring of patients with COVID-19. _Nursing Open_, _8_(6), 3538–3546. https://doi.org/10.1002/nop2.903

Khoshmehr, Z., Barkhordari-Sharifabad, M., Nasiriani, K., & Fallahzadeh, H. (2020). Moral courage and psychological empowerment among nurses. _BMC Nursing_, _19_(43). https://doi.org/10.1186/s12912-020-00435-9

Lee, S. (2017). Advancing caring literacy in practice, education, and health systems. In S. Lee, P. Palmeire, & J. Watson (Eds.), _Global advances in human caring literacy_. Springer.

Mezirow, J., & Taylor, E. (2009). _Transformative learning in practice: Insights from community, workplace, and higher education_. Jossey-Bass.

University of Auckland. (2022, May). *Curriculum structure paper*. Curriculum Framework Transformation Structure Working Group. https://www.auckland.ac.nz/en/on-campus/life-on-campus/latest-student-news/curriculum-framework-transformation-programme0/curriculum-framework-transformation-programme/structure.html

Van Schalkwyk, S. C., Hafler, J., Brewer, T. F., Maley, M. A., Margolis, C., McNamee, L., Meyer, I., Peluso, M. J., Schmutz, A. M. S., Spak, J. M., Davies, D., & Bellagio Global Health Education Initiative (2019). Transformative learning as pedagogy for the health professions: A scoping review. *Medical Education, 53*(6), 547–558. https://doi.org/10.1111/medu.13804

Wallace, C., Vidgen, R., Kirshner, S., Caetano, T., Sepasspour, R., & Weatherall, K. (2022). *Checkmate humanity: The how and why of responsible AI*. Global Stories.

Watson, J. (2017). Global advances in human caring literacy. In S. Lee, P. Palmieri, & J. Watson (Eds.), *Global advances in human caring literacy*. Springer.

Watson, J. (2018). *Unitary Caring Science: The philosophy and praxis of nursing*. University Press of Colorado.

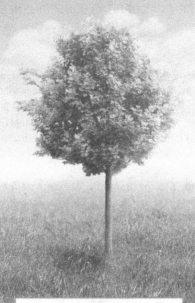

REIMAGINING REFLECTION TO DEVELOP AND SUSTAIN PERSONAL AND PROFESSIONAL PRACTICE

Gwen Sherwood, PhD, RN, FAAN, ANEF
Sara Horton-Deutsch, PhD, RN, FAAN, ANEF, SGAHN

LEARNING OBJECTIVES/SUBJECTIVES

- Examine models of reflective practice to develop and sustain personal and professional practice.

- Reimagine reflective practices for bridging real-world experiences with theory-guided learning to engage learners in practice development.

- Explore emancipatory learning by guiding nurses in connecting personal experiences with authentic being as a nurse.

- Develop tools and strategies to instill habits of reflective practice.

BEFORE YOU BEGIN

Chapter 2 explores a new vision for nursing education to develop transformative learners who cultivate self-awareness and apply a critical reasoning process that both questions actions and reassesses what is known (Day & Sherwood, 2022). The aim is to examine how reflective practices can encourage learners to engage in both formal and self-directed learning activities (Scheel et al., 2021). Reflection can facilitate transformative learning and provide guidance to foster a supportive and nurturing environment for reflective practice (Johns, 2022). In this environment, critical thinking and authentic dialogue are promoted to encourage the exchange of ideas. Critical reflection is key to transformative learning that can lead to changes in practice. Not all reflection leads to transformation; we can question things without changing anything. Transformative reflection is a change process; transformation involves or leads to a change in perspective or way of doing or acting (Van Schalkwyk et al., 2019). It is a way of solving problems that arise in practice and education. Learners need flexible and dynamic frameworks to guide their development as they move from content (knowledge) to application (practice) (Armstrong et al., 2022) and in transitioning as new graduates or new career choices (Specter et al., 2022).

Reflective practice models for developing and sustaining personal and professional practice should be an important aspect of redesigning nursing education in preparing practice-ready graduates and recreating academic-practice connections (Sherwood & Day, 2022). Reflective practice is a model of change agency that can help to uncover gaps in education and practice for improvement both collectively and at the individual level. Tools and strategies (micropractices) for instilling habits of reflective practice (Freshwater et al., 2008) are examined in the context of emancipatory learning to guide nurses in connecting personal experiences with authentic being as a nurse (Tsimane & Downing, 2020).

Academic curricula centered on competency-based education across all levels of education are more commensurate with competency assessments in practice settings (American Association of Colleges of Nursing [AACN], 2021). Redesigning pedagogical approaches (teaching) and rethinking clinical learning experiences can guide nurses in their development to consider what they know, make interpretations, and determine thoughtful action. Engagement and reflexivity bring the presence of mind to recognize potential gaps in care and thereby improve outcomes. The principles apply to individual nurses as well as to systems of care or education.

Reflective practice can be an effective learning strategy to help bridge the chasm that sits between theory and nursing as a practice-based discipline through emancipatory learning focusing on inquiry. Tanner (2006) developed a multistep model of clinical judgment—including reflection-on-action and reflection-in-action—that helps learners process information to make decisions about their work and develop clinical reasoning to "think like a nurse." It is nurses' critical thinking and analyses that provide the foundation for a practice-based discipline ready to address 21st-century health problems (Benner et al., 2010) and is reinforced as a competency statement in the Knowledge domain in the 2021 AACN Essentials (AACN, 2021).

DOMAINS FOR CORE COMPETENCIES OF PROFESSIONAL NURSING EDUCATION

The domains and descriptors used in the Essentials are listed here:

Domain 1: Knowledge for Nursing Practice Descriptor

Integration, translation, and application of established and evolving disciplinary nursing knowledge and ways of knowing, as well as knowledge from other disciplines, including a foundation in liberal arts and natural and social sciences. This distinguishes the practice of professional nursing and forms the basis for clinical judgment and innovation in nursing practice.

Domain 2: Person-Centered Care Descriptor

Person-centered care focuses on the individual within multiple complicated contexts, including family and/or important others. Person-centered care is holistic, individualized, just, respectful, compassionate, coordinated, evidence-based, and developmentally appropriate. Person-centered care builds on a scientific body of knowledge that guides nursing practice regardless of specialty or functional area.

Domain 3: Population Health Descriptor

Population health spans the healthcare delivery continuum from public health prevention to disease management of populations and describes collaborative activities with both traditional and non-traditional partnerships from affected communities, public health, industry, academia, healthcare, local government entities, and others for the improvement of equitable population health outcomes.

Domain 4: Scholarship for Nursing Discipline Descriptor

The generation, synthesis, translation, application, and dissemination of nursing knowledge to improve health and transform healthcare.

Domain 5: Quality and Safety Descriptor

Employment of established and emerging principles of safety and improvement science. Quality and safety, as core values of nursing practice, enhance quality and minimize risk of harm to patients and providers through both system effectiveness and individual performance.

Domain 6: Interprofessional Partnerships Descriptor

Intentional collaboration across professions and with care team members, patients, families, communities, and other stakeholders to optimize care, enhance the healthcare experience, and strengthen outcomes.

Domain 7: Systems-Based Practice Descriptor

Responding to and leading within complex systems of healthcare. Nurses effectively and proactively coordinate resources to provide safe, quality, equitable care to diverse populations.

Domain 8: Informatics and Healthcare Technologies Descriptor

Information and communication technologies and informatics processes are used to provide care, gather data, form information to drive decision-making, and support professionals as they expand knowledge and wisdom for practice. Informatics processes and technologies are used to manage and improve the delivery of safe, high-quality, and efficient healthcare services in accordance with best practice and professional and regulatory standards.

Domain 9: Professionalism Descriptor

Formation and cultivation of a sustainable professional nursing identity, accountability, perspective, collaborative disposition, and comportment that reflects nursing's characteristics and values.

Domain 10: Personal, Professional, and Leadership Development Descriptor

Participation in activities and self-reflection that foster personal health, resilience, well-being, lifelong learning, and the acquisition of nursing expertise and assertion of leadership.

(American Association of Colleges of Nursing, 2021).

MICROPRACTICES

1. Reflect on how nurses transition from the structured world of academic education to clinical practice. What experiences have you encountered in managing transitions:

   a. Into nursing school

   _____

   _____

   b. Into clinical practice

   _____

   _____

   c. Changing specialty areas or work units

   _____

   _____

   d. From clinical practice to educator

   _____

   _____

2. What are ways nurse educators and mentors can help learners, new graduates, or clinicians transition and adapt to new situations so they are more equipped to apply what they know in their new roles?

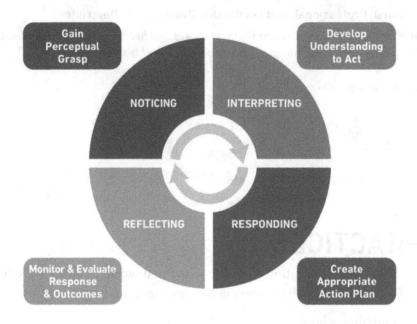

FIGURE 2.1 Clinical Judgment Model based on Tanner, 2006.

3. Reflect on a recent experience that has meaning for you. Apply Tanner's Clinical Judgment Model (2006) to identify the spectrum of critical reasoning and reflection throughout the experience. (Refer to Figure 2.1). Write about the experience using these guidelines:

a. What did you first notice? What were your observations that helped you gain a perceptual grasp?

_____

_____

b. How did you begin to interpret what was happening? How did you begin to develop understanding of the situation so you could determine actions? What knowledge, previous experiences, and understandings helped you to choose a course of action?

_____

_____

c. How did you respond? What action plan did you create? What interventions were put in place?

_____

_____

d. At the time, did you reflect on the experience to monitor and assess responses and outcomes? What changes would you instill for future situations?

_____

_____

4. Now, consider principles of transformative learning. Did you feel you experienced a change in behavior as a result of your reflecting on the structure, process, and outcomes? Describe changes in perspective.

_____

_____

LEARNING NARRATIVE

Mrs. Garcia is a 45-year-old undocumented immigrant from Nicaragua who has been diagnosed with type 2 diabetes. She has been admitted to the hospital for complications related to her diabetes, including hyperglycemia and dehydration. Her nurse, Adrianne, is responsible for Mrs. Garcia's care. Adrianne recognizes that caring for Mrs. Garcia requires a culturally sensitive approach, appreciating she may have unique cultural beliefs and practices related to health and illness. In addition, as an immigrant herself, Adrianne is aware that her pain and guilt surface when Mrs. Garcia talks about missing her family whom she cannot visit due to being undocumented. She reaches out to you, the nurse educator, to guide her in processing her emotions and in how to use the Caritas Processes to guide her in caring for Mrs. Garcia.

1. What are you most concerned about in caring for Mrs. Garcia?

_____

_____

2. What emotional support would be most helpful to Mrs. Garcia?

_____

_____

3. Choose two Caritas Processes to apply to Adrianne's care of Mrs. Garcia.

1) _____

2) _____

    a. Explain their value to Adrianne in providing care based on cultural sensitivity, competence, and caring literacy.

    _____

    _____

    b. Considering the overall learning experience, how would the Caritas Processes be part of Adrianne's reflection on the learning experience?

    _____

    _____

REFLECTIVE QUESTIONS

1. Evidence indicates many of us teach the way we were taught, which may mean we are preparing graduates for a healthcare system that no longer exists. How do the supporting theories in this chapter inform the discussion?

_____

_____

2. What are pedagogical strategies that engage learners and spark their imaginations in preparing for working in ever-changing clinical situations?

_____

_____

3. What are effective strategies as new graduates transition to the workplace?

_____

_____

4. What are ways to provide a welcoming, inclusive environment?

_____

_____

5. Describe how reflective practice enables one to examine an experience by first constructing, deconstructing, and reconstructing.

_____

_____

6. What is unique about the duality of academic and workplace learning that forms the core of nursing education within a practice-based discipline?

_____

_____

7. What is meant by saying education and practice are mirrors of each other?

_____

_____

REFERENCES

American Association of Colleges of Nursing. (2021). *The essentials: Core competencies for professional nursing education*. https://www.aacnnursing.org/Portals/42/AcademicNursing/pdf/Essentials-2021.pdf

Armstrong, G., Sherwood, G., Ironside, P., Cerbie Brown, E. & Wonder, A. (2022). Reflective practice: Using narrative pedagogy to foster quality and safety. In G. Sherwood & J. Barnsteiner (Eds.), *Quality and safety in nursing: A competency approach to improving outcomes* (3rd ed., pp. 301–320). Wiley-Blackwell.

Benner, P., Sutphen, M., Leonard, V., & Day, L. (2010). *Educating nurses: A call for radical transformation*. Jossey-Bass.

Day, L., & Sherwood, G. (2022). Transforming education to transform practice: Integrating quality and safety using unfolding case studies. In G. Sherwood & J. Barnsteiner (Eds.), *Quality and safety in nursing: A competency approach to improving outcomes* (3rd ed., pp. 269–300). Wiley-Blackwell.

Freshwater, D., Horton-Deutsch, S., Sherwood, G., & Taylor, B. (2005). *The scholarship of reflective practice* [Position paper]. Sigma Theta Tau International. http://www.nursingsociety.org/docs/default-source/position-papers/resource_reflective.pdf?sfvrsn=4.

Johns, C. (2022). *Becoming a reflective practitioner* (3rd ed.). Wiley-Blackwell.

Scheel, L. S., Bydam, J., & Peters, M. D. J. (2021). Reflection as a learning strategy for the training of nurses in clinical practice setting: A scoping review. *JBI Evidence Synthesis, 19*(12), 3268–3300. https://doi.org/10.11124/JBIES-21-00005

Sherwood, G., & Day, L. (2022). Quality and safety in clinical learning environments. In G. Sherwood & J. Barnsteiner (Eds.), *Quality and safety in nursing: A competency approach to improving outcomes* (3rd ed., pp. 321–348). Wiley-Blackwell.

Spector, N., Ulrich, B., & Barnsteiner, J. (2017). Improving quality and safety with transition to practice. In G. Sherwood & J. Barnsteiner (Eds.), *Quality and safety in nursing: A competency approach to improving outcomes* (2nd ed., pp. 281–300). Wiley-Blackwell.

Tanner, C. A. (2006). Thinking like a nurse: A research-based model of clinical judgment in nursing. *Journal of Nursing Education, 45*(6), 204–211. https://doi.org/10.3928/01484834-20060601-04

Tsimane, T., & Downing, C. (2020). A model to facilitate transformative learning in nursing education. *International Journal of Nursing Science, 7*(3), 269–276. https://doi.org/10.1016/j.ijnss.2020.04.006

Van Schalkwyk, S. C., Hafler, J., Brewer, T. F., Maley, M. A., Margolis, C., McNamee, L., Meyer, I., Peluso, M. J., Schmutz, A. M., Spak, J. M., Davies, D., & Bellagio Global Health Education Initiative. (2019). Transformative learning as pedagogy for the health professions: A scoping review. *Medical Education, 53*(6), 547–558. https://doi.org/10.1111/medu.13804

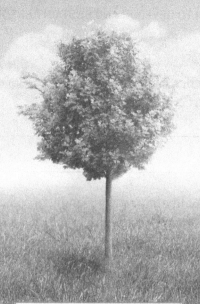

CHAPTER 3

REIMAGINING CREATIVE SPACE FOR REFLECTION IN A CARING SCIENCE PARADIGM

Anna Biley, Dip. N, MSc, Doctorate of Caring Science, Caritas Coach

LEARNING OBJECTIVES/SUBJECTIVES

- Describe the ethics and values of Watson Caring Science.

- Examine the relationship between reflective practice and Watson Caring Science.

- Analyze what it means to hold space and be in authentic presence.

- Apply the Caritas Processes to support deep listening and nurture learning communities as a safe space for reflective practice.

BEFORE YOU BEGIN

This chapter delves into Watson Caring Science and its application in nursing and healthcare. The author emphasizes the importance of care, compassion, and dignity as universal human values, constants that connect us and define who we are. The chapter explores the concept of reflection as presence and deep listening—of space and holding space for healing, reflection, and restoration.

The chapter discusses the Caritas Processes, principles and practices rooted in Watson's (2018) Theory of Human Caring. The theory emphasizes the importance of the nurse-patient relationship and the integration of caring values into healthcare practice. The Caritas Processes provide a framework for understanding and implementing caring practices in nursing and invite key questions for deep, transformative reflection and self-care. The author encourages nurses to own their vulnerability and to face their shared humanity in new ways, suggesting that in uncertain times, Caritas reflection can provide "safe space" and stability.

The concepts of authentic presence and space are explored in depth as physical, emotional, and spiritual endeavors. The chapter emphasizes the importance of being fully present for another person, creating safe space to listen deeply and explore feelings. The author suggests that creating space for reflection and healing can be achieved through various means such as art, poetry, music, journaling, or meditation.

The chapter also discusses the concept of "holding space." The author shares a personal narrative of how she applied these principles in her own life, particularly during a difficult time when her husband was dying. She emphasizes the importance of being present, holding space for caring reflection, and co-creating intentional listening.

The chapter concludes with a series of reflective questions designed to encourage readers to consider how they can apply the Caritas Processes and the principles of Caring Science in their own lives and work. Readers are invited to contemplate which Caritas Process is most relevant to their work, how they might use the Caring Science touchstones for self-care, and how they can grow and nurture a community of reflective learning.

In essence, this chapter deeply explores the principles of Caring Science and how they can be applied in nursing and healthcare to promote healing, compassion, and dignity. It encourages readers to reflect on their practices and consider how they can incorporate these principles into their lives and work.

MICROPRACTICES AND LEARNING ACTIVITIES

The WCSI Caritas Coach Education Program (CCEP) is a six-month immersion into Watson Caring Science (www.watsoncaringscience.org). In the context of loving, trusting, caring relationships, it is a process of deep sharing and personal reflection. Students (or coaches) post reflections on an internet learning platform discussion board. A dynamic connection and flow of energy emerge as all listen to and share their stories. In response to a post in which the author shared some personal, negative self-talk, a fellow coach responded, "Anna, allow yourself some grace." Those words touched my heart and were transformative in my CCEP journey and personal grief.

G.R.A.C.E. MICROPRACTICE

Here is a short meditation/micropractice. Based on the acronym G.R.A.C.E., it is a tool to cultivate compassion (www.upaya.org). Use it to find center, find stillness, and remember your authentic self:

- **G—Gather attention.** *Focus on breathing and being physically present. Still the mind. How is my body?*

- **R—Recall intention and commitment to act with integrity.** *Why am I here?*

- **A—Attune to the flow of self/other energy.** *Create gentle space, inviting a remembering. Who am I?*

- **C—Consider the wise and compassionate path.** *What do I see, sense, and learn? How may I serve?*

- **E—Engage in compassionate action.** *Acknowledge what has taken place. End the interaction by breathing, releasing, and letting go.*

Source: Halifax, 2015, p. 241; www.upaya.org

QUESTIONS FOR REFLECTION

1. What does "cultivating compassion" mean to you, and how does it manifest in your practice?

   _____

   _____

   _____

2. What does "allow yourself some grace" mean to you?

   _____

   _____

   _____

QUESTION FOR DEEPER REFLECTION

How may this microbiopractice be useful to you as a daily practice?

_____

_____

_____

MICROPRACTICE: HOLDING INTENTIONAL SPACE FOR CARING REFLECTION

Being alongside in authentic presence, we are "reminded and remember our most authentic human self and service" (Watson, 2005, p. 96) and uncover and recognize patterns that no longer serve us. Nurses spend their days holding the "tears and fears" of others (Watson, 2008, p. 102) and in doing so, create space for healing. And yet, "space is an interesting concept to ponder" (Lombard & Horton-Deutsch, 2017, p. 74). The yearning for "space" when stressed, tired, or in need of reflection and restoration is something we are all familiar with. It may manifest physically, for example in gazing at the stars or returning to a special place in nature. Space may be an emotional or spiritual endeavor of journeying inwards to find stillness and peace, perhaps through self-development microbiopractices such as art, poetry, music, journaling, or meditation (one microbiopractice you might find helpful, "G.R.A.C.E. Microbiopractice," is in the nearby sidebar). It may be some or all of these, or something unique, just for you. Whatever it is, the notion of "space" echoes a shared human experience. Explaining what it means to hold space for another, Einion (2022) states:

> To hold space means to be physically, mentally, and emotionally present for another person, creating the conditions for them to feel safe, explore their feelings, experience whatever is happening at that moment, and suspend judgment for that period of time. Regardless of what we might perceive, think, or believe about a particular situation, action, decision, or opinion, to hold space means to be lovingly present without preconditions, presuppositions, and without preconceptions. (p. 7)

The notion of "holding space" is not new. From Heidegger's philosophical perspective, "space is the medium through which relationships flow" (Lombard & Horton-Deutsch, 2017, p. 74). Offering kindness, empathic listening, sharing stories, or holding deep space for others when they can't do it for themselves are all manifestations of holding space (Plett, 2020). For millennia, humanity has held space in the life and death transition (Andrews, 2017). Midwives at the beginning and end of life, nurses, and nurturers have created deep spaces to hold each other in the rawness of our humanity, bearing witness to fear, joy, hope, loss, and broken hearts. As natural as a smile and as instinctive as a hug, holding deep space in anticipation of the first and last breath is "in our bones" (Warner, 2013, p. 32). Holding space then is intuitive (Plett, 2020). At all levels, it is what we do because we are human, because we are connected, and because "walking alongside is what you are here to do" (Biley, 2019, p. 4).

Holding space begins with loving-kindness and compassion for self (Halifax, 2015). The Caritas Processes hold this space by inviting gentle self-care and "compassion for ourselves, for others and humanity" (Horton-Deutsch & Rosa, 2019, p. 167). As unitary, interconnected beings, holding space for self is a mindful act that creates a healing environment for all (Caritas Process 8). Still, silent, and connected with our deepest sense of knowing (Caritas Process 6), holding space is an invitation to pause, breathe, listen, and "bring the mind home" (Johns, 2022, p. 23). Holding space for caring and healing in authentic caring presence, Watson (2008) detailed Caring Science touchstones as daily micropractices for reflection and presence in the beginning, middle, end, and continuing (Table 3.1).

TABLE 3.1   TOUCHSTONES: SETTING INTENTIONALITY AND CONSCIOUSNESS FOR CARING AND HEALING

CARING IN THE BEGINNING

- Begin the day with silent gratitude; set your intentions to be open to give and receive all that you are here to give and receive this day; intend to bring your full self, in the day-to-day moments of this day, cultivating a loving, caring consciousness toward yourself and all others who enter your path.

CARING IN THE MIDDLE

- Take quiet moments to "center," to empty out, to be still with yourself before entering a patient's room or when entering a meeting; cultivate a loving-caring consciousness toward each person and each situation you encounter throughout the day; make an effort "to see" who the spirit-filled person is behind the patient/colleague.

- Return to these loving-centered intentions again and again, throughout the day, helping yourself to remember why you are here.

- In the middle of stressful moments, remember to breathe; ask for guidance when unsure, confused, and frightened; forgive and bless each situation.

- Let go of that which you cannot control.

CARING IN THE END

- At the end of the day, fold these intentions into your heart; commit yourself to cultivating a loving-caring practice for yourself.

- Use whatever has presented itself to you this day as lessons to teach you to grow more deeply into your own humanity and inner wisdom.

- At the end of the day, offer gratitude for all that has entered the sacred circle of your life and work this day.

- Bless, release, and dedicate the day to a higher, deeper order of the great sacred circle of life.

CARING CONTINUING

- Create your own intentions and your own authentic presence to prepare your *Caritas Consciousness;* find your individual spiritual path toward cultivating caring consciousness and meaningful experiences in your life and work and the world.

Source: Watson, 2008, p. 51

QUESTIONS FOR PERSONAL REFLECTION

1. What parts of Watson's touchstones micropractice speak to you today?

    _____

    _____

    _____

2. As a tool for self-reflection, how can the touchstones be incorporated into your daily nursing practice?

    _____

    _____

    _____

LEARNING NARRATIVE

The following learning narrative is the author's personal experience of being alongside her husband as he lived his dying.

When my husband was first diagnosed with terminal cancer, I was offered what was to become the most helpful advice I had ever received. My brother, an intensive care nurse for many years, said to me, "Be the listener." He told me that my husband would not have the capacity to take in all the complex information thrown at us at the time. Some things were just too hard to hear. Of course, as a nurse myself I knew that, but living it when it was my life partner's death sentence was another matter. And so I learned to listen deeply. To become still. To read silence, hands, faces, and to hear the buried muffles of unspoken truths.

In the following weeks he lived his dying, and death came to us as destiny took its inevitable and heartbreaking course. Through long days and even longer nights, I held space and silence and I listened. And something began to happen. So often in the past I had doubted the authority of my own experience and yet, at the still point, at the center of the chaos that was our cancer-dominated reality, I began to hear my inner voice, telling me again and again, "You know what to do. Trust what you know." Being with dying brought to the fore the deepest human instinct to bring compassion, care, and dignity to the moment.

It is said that Caring Science starts with self. But in truth, at that time, there was no sense of self, only instinct, intuition, and a visceral calling to nurture and protect my loved ones. Over time, the inner voice became stronger and would not be silenced. Scrambling back from the abyss of bereavement in the months beyond my husband's death, safe ground slowly revealed itself, and it was there in snatched spaces of reflection that Caring Science offered a guiding hand to steady the fledgling feet of a newly anointed widow and single mum. Somehow, I had to survive because my kids needed me, and the only way I could do that was to begin caring for and listening to self.

1. How are the Caritas Processes manifest in this learning narrative?

   _____

   _____

   _____

2. Being alongside in her husband's dying, how did the author show up in authentic presence and hold space for self/other?

   _____

   _____

   _____

3. How does this narrative explore deep listening and the voice of the inner teacher?

   _____

   _____

   _____

REFLECTIVE QUESTIONS

1. You are invited to revisit and reflect on the Caritas Processes. Which one do you find most relevant to your work? Why?

   _____

   _____

   _____

2. Guided by the Caring Science touchstones described in this chapter, what self-care practices might be helpful to you?

   _____

   _____

   _____

3. How might the touchstones help you in being/becoming reflective in the moment?

_____

_____

_____

4. How might being in authentic presence, holding space, and co-creating intentional listening support you in deepening your journey of self-reflection?

_____

_____

_____

5. How can you grow and nurture a community of reflective learning?

_____

_____

_____

REFERENCES

Andrews, E. (2017). Holding space with women in the labyrinth. *Midwifery Today, 121,* 9–11.

Biley, A. (2019). *Birds hold our secrets: A Caritas story of grief and remembering.* Watson Caring Science Institute: Lotus Library.

Einion, A. (2022, February). Holding space. *Practicing Midwife, 10.*

Halifax, J. (2015). *Standing at the edge.* Flatiron Books.

Horton-Deutsch, S., & Rosa, W. (2019). Caring science and reflective practice. In W. Rosa, S. Horton-Deutsch & J. Watson (Eds.), *A handbook for caring science* (pp. 163–171). Springer.

Johns, C. (2022). *Becoming a reflective practitioner.* John Wiley & Sons, Ltd.

Lombard, K., & Horton-Deutsch, S. (2017). Creating space for reflection: The importance of presence in the teaching-learning process. In S. Horton-Deutsch & G. Sherwood, *Reflective practice: Transforming education and improving outcomes* (2nd ed., pp. 77–93). Sigma.

Plett, H. (2020). *The art of holding space.* Page Two Books.

Warner, F. (2013). *The soul midwives' handbook.* Hay House.

Watson, J. (2005). *Caring science as sacred science.* FA Davis.

Watson, J. (2008). *The philosophy and science of caring* (Revised ed.). University Press of Colorado.

Watson, J. (2018). *Unitary caring science.* University Press of Colorado.

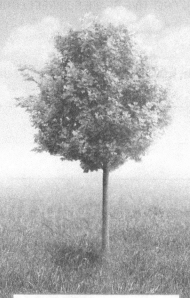

CHAPTER 4

SELF-REFLECTION THROUGH THE LENS OF UNITARY CARING SCIENCE: LEARNING TO LISTEN AND LISTENING TO LEARN

Christine Griffin, PhD, RN, NPD-BC, CPN, Caritas Coach & Leader
Sara Horton-Deutsch, PhD, RN, FAAN, ANEF, SGAHN, Caritas Coach & Leader

---

LEARNING OBJECTIVES/SUBJECTIVES

- Describe theoretical frameworks that support listening as an essential element of reflection and nursing's philosophical, moral, and ethical values.

- Explore ways to listen more deeply and wisely with others.

- Engage in individual and relational listening micropractices that serve to build and deepen the aptitude for reflection.

- Apply intentional listening to enrich personal and professional growth, enhance communication with others, and build caring-healing relationships.

BEFORE YOU BEGIN

This chapter is a deep dive into the world of reflective practice, critical thinking, and Caring Science as guides to intentional deep listening for building caring/healing relationships and personal and professional growth. The chapter empowers learners to understand themselves and others better, fostering compassion and connection and creating a supportive environment for personal growth and healing.

The chapter introduces the concept of Unitary Caring Science, a holistic approach to nursing that emphasizes self-reflection, ongoing learning, and relationship-centered care (Horton-Deutsch & Anderson, 2018; Sitzman, 2007). It expands the concept of evidence-based practice to include all forms of knowledge and invites consideration of caring literacies rather than just competencies. Caring literacies refer to ways of being and relating to others that nurses must continually cultivate (Watson, 2017).

The authors also discuss the importance of professionalism—defined by ethical behavior, accountability, and a commitment to excellence—in nursing practice. Nurses who practice from this perspective act with integrity, take accountability for their actions, and strive for excellence in all aspects of their practice.

The chapter also explores Caring Science and reflective practices in action. It provides examples of how hospitals have implemented these practices to support nursing staff, such as using touchpoints to invite staff to pause throughout their day and creating safe spaces for caregivers to share the emotional facets of being a nurse.

In the educational setting, the chapter discusses using formats such as Caritas or Healing Circle to create a safe space for learning. This approach fosters a culture of respect and understanding and creates an environment where learners are empowered to share their thoughts and ideas—and is conducive to building caring literacy, expanding ways of knowing and knowledge development, and practicing person-centered care, professionalism, and personal and professional development (Baldwin & Linnea, 2010; Griffin et al., 2021).

Micropractices include Caring Science Centering and creating sacred moments of care through pause, presence, and peace. These micropractices can be incorporated into academic and clinical settings as practices of reflection before, during, and/or after action.

In summary, this chapter is a guide to developing a deeper understanding of self and others through reflective practice, critical thinking, and Caring Science. It encourages learners to listen deeply, engage in self-reflection, and cultivate caring literacies, all of which are essential for personal and professional growth in the field of nursing.

MICROPRACTICES AND LEARNING ACTIVITIES

MICROPRACTICE: CARING SCIENCE CENTERING

- Find a quiet and comfortable place to sit or stand. Take a moment to ground yourself, placing your feet firmly on the ground and feeling the support of the earth beneath you.

- Take a deep breath through your nose, and slowly exhale through your mouth. As you exhale, release any tension or stress you may be holding in your body.

- Close your eyes or soften your gaze and recall a person or situation you care deeply about—a loved one, a patient, a friend, a pet, or a cause that you're passionate about.

- As you picture this person or situation, focus on sending them compassion, kindness, and love. Imagine wrapping them in a warm, comforting embrace and sending them positive energy and healing thoughts.

- As you continue sending compassion and love to this person or situation, extend these feelings to yourself. Know that caring for yourself is just as important as caring for others, and allow yourself to feel deserving of compassion and love.

- In this space of compassion for self and others, gently ask yourself, what gifts do I bring to this world? What can others depend on me for? What have others told me they are grateful to me for?

- As you breathe in your gifts, imagine how these gifts tie to your purpose. As a nurse, as a person, how do you want to live out this purpose?

- Take a few more deep breaths, and visualize yourself surrounded by love and care. See yourself living authentically to your unique purpose.

- When you feel ready, slowly open your eyes, and return to the present moment, carrying the feeling of love and care with you as you go about your day.

As a nurse more profoundly understands and connects to their authentic self, they can begin to build more self-care practices that keep them in the right relation with whom they are meant to be. Unitary Caring Science offers a road map for practices for self-care within the 10 Caritas Processes. While often highlighted as ways of being and becoming in response to patient needs, when practiced with self first, the nurse naturally has the inclination and capacity to offer them to the patient (Watson, 2008, 2018).

MICROPRACTICE: PAUSE, PRESENCE, PEACE

Pause: Slow down, check in with yourself, and set an intention.

Presence: Pay full attention to what is happening in the moment of care.

Peace: Set down what you can to intentionally move to the next moment of care.

LEARNING NARRATIVE

A new nurse, Maria, sees the call light go off in a patient's room and gets up to respond. This patient, Victor, was traveling from South Africa to find a medical solution for an ongoing and debilitating health crisis. It is just he and his mother who made the journey because of finances. Another nurse on the unit remarks, "Beware. I just saw the patient's mom enter the room. You know what happened last time she was here." Maria enters the room to find the mother of her 25-year-old patient standing next to the enteral feeding pump and bag. Before Maria can say anything, the mother, who understands English but speaks with a deep accent, begins to yell that she has found some dirt on the inside of the feeding bag. She yells that Maria is incompetent and is trying to harm her son. She demands to see the manager of the unit and wants to fire Maria immediately. Maria knows that what appears to be dirt inside the bag is a new ferrous sulfate supplement ordered this morning and added to the feeding before the family had arrived. Maria quickly explains this to the mother, but the anger doesn't subside; it only heightens her resolve to explain that the bag is dirty and that no one cares that her son is receiving dirty food, that this is not the first time she has complained about the food, and how no one on this unit cares about her son until she gets angry and demands it. After several minutes of hearing insults and shouldering all the anger, Maria decides to leave the room. She finds the charge nurse to explain that the mother would like a different nurse. The charge nurse explains that it is not possible to change assignments at the moment, but when she has time, she will go into the room and talk with the patient and family to try and smooth things out. Twenty minutes later, the call light goes off again, and the mother demands to see Maria immediately. Maria is standing outside of the room, knowing that the charge nurse has not been in yet, and is trying to find the courage to open the door.

1. Imagine what would be running through your mind if you are in this nurse's shoes. What is your intention when you enter this room for the second time, carrying with you the first experience? How deep does the hurt go for you? How do you prepare yourself to open the door?

2. Notice if your first thoughts are to be able to explain, rationalize, or set the record straight with the mother. Are there parts of you that want to be heard? Do you want to convince the mother that you and the other nurses care about all the patients? Does letting this moment go unresolved diminish you in any way or affect your ability to care authentically?

Now imagine using the practices we reviewed in this chapter to inform and repattern the potential outcomes of this scenario. Notice we say *potential outcomes* because even when we show up as the best versions of ourselves, we cannot control the response of others. The practices of Unitary Caring Science help us understand that when the best version of ourselves show up, the outcome is secondary. What matters is authentically living out who we are meant to be, making the unique difference we are called to make, and having peace within knowing that we did not contribute to reducing another human being in any way. No simple ask, especially when you are asked to do this while others may fail. This is why nursing is not just a profession; it is a calling. It is why Jean Watson says nursing sustains another until they can do it for themselves.

1. Apply the practices of pause, presence, and peace to repattern this experience.

2. What is a meaningful pause you can take before entering a patient room that could be filled with tension? Think about what you might need to do first to care for yourself. Perhaps take a breath, talk it over with a fellow nurse, get a drink of water, or let them know you will be in in a few minutes so you can gather your thoughts.

3. What intention do you want to set before entering this room? Perhaps it is the ability to listen deeply without needing to correct what is said. Perhaps it is a practice of equanimity, where you set an intention not to own any negativity and keep an internal boundary of what you accept as fact vs. perception. Perhaps you intend to infuse the environment with dignity for everyone, including yourself, so that you know when it is time to listen, respond, and step away if necessary.

4. What will you need to stay present with the patient and the mother? Is there a practice you know can help you settle in? Does it help to ask them to sit down with you? Do you need permission to take notes, so you capture everything? What will you do if you find you are distracted? How will you reset or re-center yourself?

5. How will you work to find the peace you need after this experience? Will you take a few moments to process this? Will you find another nurse and ask them to listen to you? Will you allow yourself space in the moment to set it down and set an intention to talk it out or write about it later?

Now imagine a Unitary Caring Science approach to this scenario.

As Maria stands at the door, she takes a moment to pause and take a deep breath. She reflects on the words the mother had said about her son's food being dirty and wonders what that meant to this mother. She imagines that if she walked into a room of a loved one and assumed the care was subpar, how vulnerable, guilty, and out of control that would make her feel. She looks beyond the words and imagines what it would be like to be in a foreign place with language and cultural differences and tries to imagine being trusting and at ease within those barriers. Maria sets an intention of listening to this mother with the only intention of helping her suffer less at this moment—to ease her burden and make sure the mother can feel this nurse's authentic presence and care.

As she opens the door, the mother points to the pump and remarks coldly that it was beeping and that maybe Maria can at least manage that. She then asks when another nurse will take over her son's care. Maria notices that she needs to reset after hearing this remark and takes a nice slow breath to remember her intention. She asks the mom if this was an okay time for them to talk and invites her to sit down with her in the window seating area. Reluctantly, the mother joins her. Maria praises the mother for fighting so hard for her son's care and tells her she admires how much she loves him. Then she asks if she could help her understand what she meant when she said that her son was receiving dirty food. This gives the mother permission to explain that in their home, they could not always afford the best food for their large family. They often had to resort to buying food that wasn't fresh or past the expiration date, sometimes even using the scraps of other people's meals to feed themselves. She said that she believes this is why her son is having so many difficulties and blames herself for his poor health. Within minutes, Maria can now see a bigger picture of pain, guilt, and the redemption this mother needs. While not excusing the behavior, it gives a new lens to process it through. Maria then asks the mother what she needs to trust the nurses taking care of her son. The patient's mother shares that the food is always prepared outside the room, so she never sees the packages or process, and she imagines that because they are from another country, they are not getting the same as other patients. Maria shows the mother where the food is stored, how new feeding bags are opened, and what safeguards are in place to ensure the enteral food was prepared to the highest of standards. The mother had no idea how many steps had happened before the pump was brought into the room.

After the shift, Maria sits quietly in her car before driving home. She allows herself to reflect on all the events of the day and her experiences within them. With just one patient, she felt a continuum of emotions from frustration and fear to compassion and understanding. Each emotion required something from her, and she notices that she was physically and emotionally drained. She then reflects on the ways she showed up that she was proud of and the real moments when her ego and survival brain took over. Overall, she is proud of herself for the courage she found to go back into the patient's room and the new perspective she learned by setting the intention of dignity. She does a practice to set down the shift and, as usual, turns on some loud music to sing her way home and let go of being a nurse so she could also be human. The next shift, Maria notices that she has this patient again and finds herself looking forward to seeing the patient, Victor, and his fierce mother.

REFLECTIVE QUESTIONS

1. How well do I listen to others? Assess your listening skills and attention to the other's words, tone, and body language.

    _____

    _____

    _____

2. How do I process and reflect on what I hear from others? Examine an interaction to assess how you take time to pause and reflect on what was said or quickly move on to the next topic. What steps can I take to deepen my reflective practice and become a more intentional listener?

    _____

    _____

    _____

3. Recall an encounter. What are my assumptions about the person I am listening to, and how might these assumptions impact my ability to hear and understand what they are truly saying?

    _____

    _____

    _____

4. How do I respond to difficult or uncomfortable conversations? How do I stay present and engaged, even when the conversation is challenging?

    _____

    _____

    _____

5. How can the 10 Caritas Processes guide me in listening and responding?

    _____

    _____

    _____

6. What micropractices can I use to improve my listening skills and stay fully present in conversations? How can I practice listening to others in more mindful, attentive, aware, and empathetic ways?

_____

_____

_____

REFERENCES

Baldwin, C., & Linnea, A. (2010). *The circle way: A leader in every chair.* Berrett-Koehler.

Griffin, C., Oman, K. S., Ziniel, S. I., Kight, S., Jacobs-Lowry, S., & Givens, P. (2021). Increasing the capacity to provide compassionate care by expanding knowledge of caring science practices at a pediatric hospital. *Archives of Psychiatric Nursing, 35*(1), 34–41. https://doi.org/10.1016/j.apnu.2020.10.019

Horton-Deutsch, S., & Anderson, J. (2018). *Caritas coaching: A journey toward transpersonal caring for informed moral action in healthcare.* Sigma.

Sitzman, K. (2007). Teaching-learning professional learning based on Jean Watson's Theory of Human Caring. *International Journal of Human Caring, 11*(4), 16–18. https://doi.org/10.20467/1091-5710.11.4.8

Watson, J. (2008). *Nursing: The philosophy and science of caring* (Rev. ed.). University of Colorado Press.

Watson, J. (2018). *Unitary caring science: The philosophy and praxis of nursing.* University of Colorado Press.

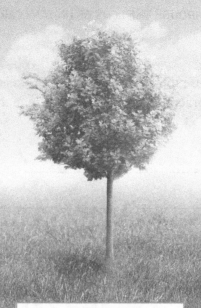

CHAPTER 5

DEEPENING OUR FOUNDATIONS: REIMAGINING OURSELVES, REIMAGINING NURSING IDENTITY

Gwen Sherwood, PhD, RN, FAAN, ANEF
Meg Moorman, PhD, RN, CNE, ANEF
Crystal Morales, MS, BSN, RN

LEARNING OBJECTIVES/SUBJECTIVES

- Develop reflective practices for attending to self as nurse for increasing self-awareness.

- Cultivate strategies for renewal in contributing to healthy work environments that promote well-being.

- Catalyze development of organizational well-being programs to reimagine emotional and organizational support in managing the intensity of nurses' work.

- Reimagine nurses' education and development based on Unitary Caring Science for sustaining well-being and growth over their professional career.

- Foster well-being for thriving in post-pandemic healing.

BEFORE YOU BEGIN

Chapter 5 deepens the foundations of what it is to be nurse, explores reflective pedagogies addressing nursing as a practice-based discipline, and includes tools and micropractices addressing self-care, wellness, and person-centered care. Reflective practices are a way to reconceptualize the full potential of what it is to be a nurse, to care for and to be cared for.

Grounded in the consciousness and clarity of Unitary Caring Science, a relational ontology of connectedness and belonging moves humanity towards a moral community where we care for self and others (Watson, 2016). Focusing on biomedical-technical science with a separatist worldview focuses on task orientation, lacking the human element of nursing and healthcare, which exacts an emotional and physical toll on nurses (Watson, 2016). Integrating Unitary Caring Science as the foundation for the discipline of nursing provides a road map for interpersonal practice where there is both being and doing, transforming healthcare with a relational way of being that sustains our shared humanity.

The concepts and practices of Unitary Caring Science are a guide for revisioning work environments for creating and sustaining nurses' well-being through "attention to self as nurse." Caring for self is a way of finding restoration from the physical and emotional demands within nursing. As essential healthcare team members in the COVID-19 pandemic, nurses' personal and professional reservoirs of strength and sustenance were tested. The chapter provides resources for reimagining self as nurse through reflective practices derived from narrative inquiry, mindful practice (Horton-Deutsch & Horton, 2003), and appreciative inquiry in developing emotional intelligence—and reflective practices applied to self-care that cultivate relationships through consciousness of self, others, and the context of practice for improving how we work and grow together (Horton-Deutsch & Sherwood, 2008).

Nurses learn and grow throughout their careers, a mark of professionalism. Transitioning to practice is aided by professional identity formation developed as part of nurses' formal education (Rasmussen et al., 2021). Habits of questioning help nurses continually examine and develop insights into the real-world nurse role and ease the transition to practice (Patel & Metersky, 2021). Content-based formal learning helps develop knowledge and skills, but nurses still must assimilate the norms, values, and attitudes that guide "thinking like a nurse" and help make sense of practice, and simultaneously develop their own self-care practices. Reflective practice guides learning from experience by considering what we know, believe, and value within the context of an event. Situated in complex environments, learners, nurses, and educators may employ reflective practices for systematically working to make sense of the whole in sustainable ways across one's professional journey; the continuing journey helps us evaluate our contributions, leading to greater satisfaction and sense of purpose in our work.

Developing reflective practice is a lifelong journey that supports and sustains career development. Reflection helps clarify how we work according to our mission and purpose and as such guides us in developing spiritual resources for managing and balancing our personal and professional lives (Willis & Sheehan, 2019).

Micropractices throughout the chapter offer ways individuals and organizations can foster nurses' well-being by guiding sense-making, resolving contradictions, and promoting professional development so nurses can experience restoration, renewal, and regeneration (Della Bella et al., 2022).

MICROPRACTICES

When new to a work culture, nurses, educators, and learners are confounded trying to absorb the social and political contexts and integrate into the professional practice framework. To instill the habit of inquiry, nurses may use reflection-on-action (see Chapter 2) for sense-making. Figure 5.1 illustrates how reflecting on practice leads to understanding experience to incorporate lessons into changes in work, contributing to personal and professional growth in continuous cycles of reflection on action.

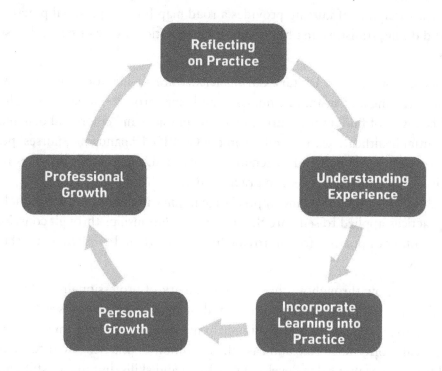

FIGURE 5.1   Reflecting for personal and professional growth.
Source: Adapted from Patel and Metersky (2021)

MICROPRACTICE: APPRECIATIVE INQUIRY

Appreciative inquiry is a positive change process to consider how to work with others by thinking of times that have worked well. Narrative approaches fit well with appreciative inquiry guided by reflective questions. Think about an experience you had with your coworkers that went well, and respond to the following guided questions:

1. What happened?

   _____

   _____

2. How do I make sense of the situation?

_____

_____

3. What was meaningful?

_____

_____

4. What questions did I ask, and how did I ask them in a person-centered way?

_____

_____

5. When and how did I know I had connected with the other person?

_____

_____

6. How can I do it again to make it an integral part of my practice?

_____

_____

MICROPRACTICE: MAKING SENSE OF A DIFFICULT DAY

Illustrating this process, Dearmin (2000) describes a micropractice on the value of reflection in making sense of practice and handling the stress of a particularly difficult day to sort out the "good and the bad bits of the day and the whole situation" (p. 163). Reflect on a day in which you felt particularly challenged. Use these three questions for analyzing the event:

1. What did I do?

_____

_____

2. What should I have done that I did not do?

_____

_____

3. How would I act differently next time?

_____

_____

MICROPRACTICE: USING VISUAL THINKING STRATEGIES FOR REFLECTIVE LEARNING

Select artwork that reflects diverse content, such as cultural differences or racial issues that represent situations nurses may find difficult to openly discuss. Analyzing artwork allows others to speak up, promotes sharing diverse views, and demonstrates educational scaffolding as participants add their perspectives (Moorman, 2017). A Visual Thinking Strategies facilitator gathers the group and asks them to spend a few moments looking at the work of art. The facilitator asks the group:

"What is going on in this painting?"

As a person responds, the facilitator will ask, "What are you seeing that makes you say that?"

After responding, the facilitator will paraphrase back what the participant said, then ask the group, "What else can we find?"

After each person has an opportunity to contribute, the facilitator can ask, "What was the correct answer?" (Groups will note that there is no one right answer and that each person's interpretation was honored and respected.)

Follow-up question: How can you use this in your nursing? What did you notice about how the group responded?

This debriefing can help to discuss a cultural scenario together, listen to each other, and demonstrate the value of multiple perspectives.

And finally: How does this apply in your work? What situations would benefit from multiple perspectives?

MICROPRACTICE: STRATEGIES FOR CREATING WELL-BEING

Challenges are a universal experience. To manage stress for daily renewal and well-being, everyone needs habits of self-care, covering a range of activities:

- Set boundaries and realize that "No" is a complete sentence!
- Take care of the physical self through exercise, nutrition, relaxation techniques, and sleep hygiene.

- Use attitude adjustment strategies such as spiritual care practices, social encounters, positive self-talk, or connecting with people who encourage healthy habits and positive attitudes.

- Maintain a gratitude journal to promote a positive attitude; use reflective prompts such as recording three good things that happened on your shift, or three things you are grateful for today. Reflect on the balance of satisfaction of fulfilling work duties and the personal cost to be able to make changes as appropriate.

- Appreciate your strengths by reducing negative self-talk, instead talking to yourself as you would to someone you love.

- Normalize responses to difficult situations.

- Recognize and seek what you truly need to be effective in your work.

- Reduce guilt and let go of the "tyranny of the shoulds." When you feel the "should" creeping in, ask yourself:

  - Does this really matter to me?

  - Do I have the energy for this right now?

- Focus your energy on things you have control over, provide input where you have influence, and learn to ignore and accept that there are things that you can neither control nor influence.

- Be a part of creating a supportive, caring work environment by providing social support to coworkers.

MICROPRACTICE: PEER SUPPORT GROUPS

Offering one-on-one peer support during high-stress times or scheduling group debriefings using a common process to guide discussion in productive communication can reduce whining or gripe sessions.

- Peer support may include statements such as:

  - "I will sit here with you."

  - "Can I call someone for you?"

  - "You don't have to do this alone."

- Reassuring statements may include:

  - "You are not alone."

  - "I understand why you might feel that way."

  - "You are going to get through this, but it will take time."

Peer support also means there are things not to say! Do not be overly reassuring or dismissive of someone's dissonance.

- Do not use platitudes such as:
  - "These things happen."
  - "It could always be worse."
  - "You know this always happens in this place."

MICROPRACTICE: FISHBOWL CHECK-IN FOR GROUP DEBRIEFING OF AN EXPERIENCE

Many events nurses experienced during the COVID-19 pandemic challenged nurses' usual way of delivering care or education. Convene a group with common goals (unit teams, study groups, clinical groups, faculty teams, etc.). Identify an event representing an area of concern that changed the usual way of accomplishing the group's mission and led to distress, unanticipated outcome, or ethical dilemmas. Use the reflective guide to process the situation to make sense of the way forward or to reach consensus. The goal is to better understand the why and not the who.

- What is the context of where and when it happened?
- What happened?
- Why was it significant?
- What concerns were there at the time?
- What was the thinking and feeling at the time and afterward?
- What choices were made and why?
- What else could have happened if other choices had been made?
- How can we prepare for future events?

LEARNING NARRATIVE

Attending to self: Using the art of clay to deepen our foundation (adapted from Parker, 1994).

Purpose: Practice mindfulness through stillness as a personal growth strategy to focus on self in wholeness, who you are as person and nurse, to support and encourage reflection on values, attitudes, beliefs, and renew your state of being.

Premise: Aesthetic expression leads us into "inner knowing places," into our creative connection within our self, and expands our situational awareness.

Method: Alone or with participants, sit quietly with soft, unobtrusive music in the background. Hold a piece of clay in your hands to begin to warm it to a softened state. Then work with the clay in any way you want—kneading it, opening, circling, pinching, or pounding—simply be in the moment. Clear any preconceived notions or barriers about creating art. Shaping the clay is getting in touch with yourself working from inside out. Breathe slowly, in and out, using principles of reflection, go into a place within yourself where you reach beyond to transcend to your undiscovered affective dimensions, often crowded by the rational self.

Reflection: The aliveness of clay as an organic, natural matter emerges into a form; meaning emerges into consciousness. Listen to your inner voice as you come out of the shaping experience. What is surfacing from your soul? How does this experience address spiritual needs?

Share with others in the group.

Write your experience as a critical reflection, a poem, or other narration to enhance the feelings of spiritual renewal and self-awareness in meeting realities around you.

_____

_____

_____

_____

REFLECTIVE QUESTIONS

1. What are ways you commit to cultivating renewal for self-care?

_____

_____

2. What are three ways your workplace can offer peer-to-peer support?

_____

_____

3. How can you help catalyze development of a well-being focus on your work environment?

_____

_____

4. How can organizations offer support for new graduates transitioning to practice, facilitating first-year integration to reduce turnover?

_____

_____

5. What are steps in designing a group session for debriefing critical incidents as part of a unit well-being initiative?

_____

_____

REFERENCES

Dearmin, N. (2000). The legacy of reflective practice. In S. Burns & C. Bulman (Eds.), *Reflective practice in nursing: The growth of the professional practitioner* (2nd ed., pp. 156–172). Blackwell Science.

Della Bella, V., Fiorini, J., Gioiello, G., Zaghini, F., & Sili, A. (2022). Towards a new conceptual model for nurses' organizational well-being: An integrative review. *Journal of Nursing Management, 30*(7), 2833–2844. https://doi.org/10.1111/jonm.13750

Horton-Deutsch, S. L., & Horton, J. M. (2003). Mindfulness: Overcoming conflict. *Archives of Psychiatric Nursing, 17*(4), 186–193.

Horton-Deutsch, S., & Sherwood, G. (2008). Reflection: An educational strategy to develop emotionally competent nurse leaders. *Journal of Nursing Management, 16*(8), 946–954. https://doi.org/10.1111/j.1365-2834.2008.00957.x

Moorman, M. (2017). The use of visual thinking strategies and art to help nurses find their voices. *Creative Nursing, 23*(3), 167–171. https://doi.org/10.1891/1078-4535.23.3.167

Parker, M. (1994). The healing art of clay: A workshop for remembering wholeness. In D. A. Gaut & A. Boykin (Eds.), *Caring as healing: Renewal through hope* (pp. 35–145). National League for Nursing Press.

Patel, K. M., & Metersky, K. (2021). Reflective practice in nursing: A concept analysis. *International Journal of Nursing Knowledge, 33*(3), 180–187. https://doi.org/10.1111/2047-3095.12350

Rasmussen, P., Henderson, A., McCallum, J., & Andrew, N. (2021). Professional identity in nursing: A mixed method research study. *Nurse Education in Practice, 52*, 103039. https://doi.org/10.1016/j.nepr.2021.103039

Watson, J. (2016). Human caring literacy. In S. Lee, P. Palmieri, & J. Watson (Eds.), *Global advances in human caring literacy* (pp. 3–11). Springer Publishing Company.

Willis, D., & Sheehan, D. (2019). Spiritual knowing: Another pattern of knowing in the discipline. *Advances in Nursing Science, 42*(1), 58–68. https://doi.org/10.1097/ANS.0000000000000236

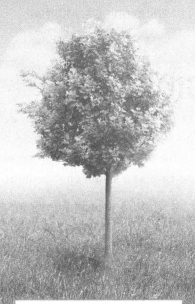

CHAPTER 6

THE ROLE OF REFLECTION IN GUIDING THE EVOLUTION OF CARE, COMPASSION, AND SOCIAL CHANGE

Erica Hooper, DNP, RN, CNL, CNS, PHN
Sara Horton-Deutsch, PhD, RN, FAAN, ANEF, SGAHN

LEARNING OBJECTIVES/SUBJECTIVES

- Examine reflective practice skills and strategies for expanding the capacity for compassionate care for self and others.

- Explore theoretical frameworks that guide care and compassion for self, others, community, and society.

- Demonstrate the value of personal experiences and stories as an inner teacher for guiding personal and professional development.

- Prioritize habits of self-care and self-compassion as the foundation to authentically care for others.

- Recognize the necessity of creating safe learning spaces as the foundation for brave learning spaces central to social change.

BEFORE YOU BEGIN

This chapter, written by Erica Hooper and Sara Horton-Deutsch, delves into the importance of reflective practice, critical thinking, and Caring Science in the field of nursing. The authors assert that these elements are crucial not only for the personal development of nursing professionals but also for the evolution of compassionate care and social change within the nursing profession.

Reflective practice is presented as a key tool for promoting compassionate care and improving systems that may hinder such practices. The authors emphasize that reflection is foundational for nursing students as they develop their professional practice. Reflective skills aim to improve self-awareness, enhance well-being, and develop resilience. Journaling is highlighted as an effective reflective practice beneficial for both novice learners and experienced professionals.

The chapter reviews Jean Watson's theory of Unitary Caring Science (2021), which provides a model for creating caring, healing environments that build human connections and break down barriers leading to inequities and injustice. This model is explicated through the 10 Caritas Processes that focus on developing a caring relationship, being compassionate, using creative problem-solving, promoting self-care and growth, creating a healing environment, assisting with basic needs, engaging in spiritual practices, promoting positive and loving interactions, using reflective practice, and honoring the unique individuality of each patient.

The authors further explore the concept of self-compassion as developed by Kristen Neff (2011). Self-compassion involves three main components: mindfulness, common humanity, and self-kindness. Mindfulness means being aware of our thoughts and feelings without judgment or criticism, while common humanity recognizes that all human beings experience suffering and struggle in life. Self-kindness involves treating ourselves with warmth, empathy, and forgiveness.

Importantly, this chapter emphasizes the necessity of educators creating secure environments for learning to ensure learners' comfort and support during their educational journey. When learners feel secure, their involvement in the learning process increases, enabling them to embrace personal and professional growth by taking risks. Safe learning spaces not only cultivate a sense of community among learners but also promote collaboration and the sharing of ideas. Progressing from safe to courageous learning spaces involves the creation of an atmosphere that not only guarantees physical and emotional safety but also motivates learners to venture outside their comfort zones, question their assumptions, and address their biases (Plett, 2020). This transition necessitates a shift from a culture that emphasizes compliance to one that values creativity, innovation, and experimentation.

Micropractices in this chapter include a personal storytelling paper; the DEAL Assignment (Ash & Clayton, 2009), which can be adapted and used as a discussion assignment; a self-care log for learners to complete over a selected period; and a reflection on the American Nurses Association (ANA) Racial Reckoning Statement (2021).

In conclusion, the chapter underscores the importance of reflective practice, critical thinking, and Caring Science in nursing. It emphasizes the need for institutional support in academic and practice settings to promote a culture of caring and compassion, fulfilling the Institute for Healthcare Improvement Quadruple Aim. By prioritizing reflective practices and recognizing their crucial role in promoting compassionate care, we can help ensure that nursing remains a discipline and profession that places care and compassion at the forefront of its practice, elevating the experience of both the care receiver and caregiver.

MICROPRACTICES

MICROPRACTICE: DEAL

Hooper and Horton-Deutsch (2023) scaffold a personal experience/storytelling paper in their wellness course to evaluate health professions students' personal/professional development and mastery of course content. The critical reflection paper invites learners to share their personal/professional experiences through the Describe, Examine, and Articulate Learning (DEAL) model (Ash & Clayton, 2009). The DEAL assignment can be used in multiple ways—for personal/professional development, civic engagement, or academic advancement—and has established psychometrics and a rubric. For the authors' purposes, students write the Describe at the beginning of the semester and complete the Examine and Articulate Learning at the end of the semester where they have the opportunity to incorporate course readings and insights gained throughout the semester.

DEAL

DEAL (Describe, Examine, and Articulate Learning) is different from your typical academic paper. It should be written in the first person. It is an opportunity to tell your story. You will write the Describe for this assignment and the Examine and Articulate Learning at the end of the semester. Using APA format (include a cover page), write a three to four page paper in response to the following:

I. DESCRIBE: Think of a time when you, a friend, a family member, or a patient you cared for were ill and how caring influenced healing. Write the narrative/story of the experience. *This should be a three to four-page thick description of the experience. You might read a thick description in a novel where the author provides details that connect you to your senses. Note: This is your story—once you start writing, it will flow, just like you are telling your friend the details of an event. This should not take much time—we want this to come from your heart.*

Now give the experience a name. The name should reflect the experience.

Name of the experience_____.

For example, Jane might name her story of using Reiki to care for her chronic pain The Power of Energy Healing.

During the final week of the semester, you will add three to four pages to the original paper through the addition of Examine and Articulate Learning sections. Begin by rereading your original paper. Now write a response using the following prompts as your inspiration (be sure to reference your two textbooks and at least one additional reading and add a reference page for the paper).

II. EXAMINE (to look closely for the purpose of learning) in fair detail the following questions. *Where you see a blank, insert the name you gave the experience. The purpose of this is to externalize the experience for examination purposes as well as deconstruct (critique dominant understandings of a particular topic—in this example, we are looking at illness).*

If _____ could talk to me, what would it say to me? For example: What would it say if The Power of Energy Healing could talk to me?

What are the main themes related to _____ embedded in the narrative?

What does _____ have you thinking about wellness practices to support healing?

What does _____ have you doing about wellness practices?

Does _____ encourage ethics/values about wellness practices?

Now, reflect on your answers and write a reflective summary statement.

III. ARTICULATE LEARNING: Respond to the following questions.

What did I learn? About myself? Healing? What I thought I thought? Etc.

How did I learn it? (Be specific. It is not sufficient to merely state what you reflected or wrote.)

Think about what it was regarding the assignment, afterward conversation, reflection, etc. that prompted your learning.

Why does it matter (personally and professionally)?

What will I do in the future, in light of it (personally and professionally)?

When you've completed your assignment, attach your Word doc for review.

MICROPRACTICE: SELF-CARE PLAN

From the authors' experiences, learners are often hard on themselves and push themselves to be the best, causing them to strengthen their inner critic. Self-criticism can be especially damaging when combined with the stress and pressure of nursing school, as student performance and overall well-being can be impacted by negative self-talk and self-doubt. These negative habits can carry over into the nursing profession if students are not prepared to better manage their stress. To maximize positive transition, nursing students need to recognize when their inner critic is being overly harsh and develop strategies to pause, reflect, and manage their stress and anxiety.

Introducing and guiding learners in self-care and compassion is a useful way to model the importance of improving self-care and weakening the inner critic to reduce stress and anxiety while in school and across their professional careers. During their wellness course, the authors introduce and allow students to complete a self-care plan to emphasize that care and compassion for self are the foundation for caring for others (Hooper & Horton-Deutsch, 2023).

SELF-CARE PLAN

In the boxes below, write your self-care goals in support of the wellness of your mind, body, and spirit. Write your goals using the S.M.A.R.T. (specific, measurable, attainable, realistic, and time-oriented) format. An example would be: Starting this Sunday I will walk in the park for 30 minutes every day of the week.

My goal to support my physical wellness is:

My goal to support my mental wellness is:

My goal to support my spiritual wellness is:

It is important to identify what may be helpful and what may be a challenge to the attainment of your goals so that you may be more focused on what you need to do to meet your goals.

The following are barriers to achieving my self-care goals (e.g., being tired at the end of the day):

1.

2.

3.

The following are helpful to achieving my self-care goals (e.g., going to the gym with a friend):

1.

2.

3.

By meeting my self-care goals, I hope to_____ (e.g., feel more peaceful):

1.

2.

3.

MICROPRACTICE: MOVING FROM SAFE TO BRAVE LEARNING SPACES TO GUIDE SOCIAL CHANGE

Professional identity formation begins by developing therapeutic relationships expressed in empathy, care, and compassion. Academic nursing programs have a responsibility to model a culture of care and compassion for their learners as they grow in professional identity and professionalism (American Association of Colleges of Nursing, 2021). A culture of care requires fostering inclusivity and diversity and begins addressing previous harm within the profession. On July 12, 2022, ANA released the formal Racial Reckoning Statement, which is the association's first step in acknowledging past actions that have negatively impacted nurses of color and perpetuated systemic racism. The Journey of Racial Reconciliation is the name for ANA's racial reckoning journey. Read the ANA Social Reckoning Statement (2021) and respond to the reflective practice questions that follow. Statement available at the following link: https://www.nursingworld.org/practice-policy/workforce/racism-in-nursing/RacialReckoningStatement/

- In what ways do I contribute to and/or not contribute to perpetuating the cycle of racism in nursing?

_____

_____

_____

_____

- How can I heal the impact of racism in nursing on myself and others?

_____

_____

_____

_____

- How can caring for myself support me to hold space for listening to others share their experiences of racism in nursing?

_____

_____

_____

_____

LEARNING NARRATIVE

Jackie is a 20-year-old BSN nursing student who has recently started the fourth year of her program. She is one month into her semester and already feeling sleep deprived, malnourished, stressed, and anxious. This semester Jackie is pleased to be taking a wellness course designed to support her learning to develop self-compassion and to take better care of herself. These concepts are new to Jackie; many of the reflective course assignments feel foreign. However, Jackie realizes she needs to change her habits and begins to incorporate new methods for thriving in school.

Jackie is relieved that her course faculty have given her permission to care for herself, as she has been so focused throughout school on caring for others, learning new skills, and passing her exams. In her wellness course she has completed a few reflection assignments emphasizing care and compassion, and she is feeling both intrigued and curious. For the first time, Jackie has become self-aware of her inner critic that often insults her worth and makes her feel bad when she doesn't get the perfect grade. She has just been given an assignment to develop a self-care plan for how she is going to care for her mind, body, and spirit over the rest of the semester. She is not sure where to begin but knows she needs to make a change to be more caring and compassionate with herself.

REFLECTIVE QUESTIONS

1. In what ways does the practice of self-care and self-compassion allow one to better care for others?

_____

_____

_____

_____

2. How does reflective practice serve as a guide for care and compassion in one's personal and professional life?

_____

_____

_____

_____

3. What do students need to learn in nursing educational programs about reflection, self-care, and self-compassion as a means for social change in nursing?

_____

_____

_____

_____

REFERENCES

American Nurses Association. (2021, June 11). *Journey of racial reconciliation: Racial reckoning statement.* https://www.nursingworld.org/practice-policy/workforce/racism-in-nursing/RacialReckoningStatement/

Ash, S., & Clayton, P. (2009). Generating, deepening, and documenting learning: The power of critical reflection in applied learning. *Journal of Applied Learning in Higher Education, 1, Fall,* 25–48.

Hooper, E., & Horton-Deutsch, S. (2023). Integrating compassion and theoretical premises of Caring Science into undergraduate health professions education. *Creative Nursing, 29*(1), 1–10.

Neff, K. (2011). *The proven power of being kind to yourself: Self-compassion.* HarperCollins.

Plett, H. (2020). *The art of holding space: A practice of love, liberation, and leadership.* Page Two.

Watson, J. (2021). *Caring science as sacred science* (Rev. Ed). Lotus Library.

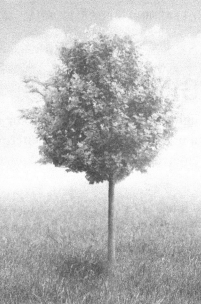

SHARING OUR STORIES: CO-CREATING LEARNING THROUGH NARRATIVE PEDAGOGY, SILENCE, AND LISTENING

Carole Hemmelgarn, MS
Gail Armstrong, PhD, DNP, ACNS-BC, RN, CNE, FAAN
Gwen Sherwood, PhD, RN, FAAN, ANEF

LEARNING OBJECTIVES/SUBJECTIVES

- Describe theoretical models for implementing various forms of narrative pedagogy.

- Demonstrate reflective practices guiding the healthcare team in learning from narratives and developing self-awareness.

- Examine the power of stories in co-creating person-centered care.

- Explore reflective practices in building authentic connections using the dynamics of listening and silence.

BEFORE YOU BEGIN

Chapter 7 emphasizes learning through silence and listening as key aspects of narrative pedagogy. The chapter explores developing and practicing listening and interpretative skills to revision how to work together, co-produce person-centered care, and enhance how we understand the context of our environment.

This chapter emphasizes ways to integrate story into both formal and informal learning in any setting. Story is a powerful learning tool because it can present a variety of evidence, personal interactions, patient voices, and varied perspectives in weaving together the narrative components of the story itself (Boykin & Schoenhofer, 1991). The chapter provides multiple models and theories that guide the use of story as a primary form of narrative pedagogy (Ironside et al., 2017). Using stories is an interactive experiential educational strategy supported by transformative learning theory. Stories illustrate knowledge application in bridging theory (knowledge) with experiences (Alteren, 2019).

There is no one way to use stories for learning. Reflective practices, however, are a vital component of how we analyze, interpret, and respond to stories and narratives (Choperena et al., 2019). While we cite stories as an example of narrative pedagogy, there are multiple forms of narratives used educationally such as case studies, problem-based learning, simulation, and team-based learning (Armstrong et al., 2022). Stories stand out as narrative by including personal aspects rather than an objective case study (Charon, 2004).

Two essential components of story are listening and context (Rockwell et al., 2022). Listening is an essential skill in learning from stories; stories require a listener, yet we rarely focus on developing this skill (Caspersz & Stasinska, 2015). Context sets the details of what is going on, defines story participants, and informs analysis and interpretation.

Numerous examples of learning through story illustrate integration of specific content such as quality and safety, clinical content, or personal and professional development. Stories from the COVID-19 pandemic illustrate how stories help nurses manage moral distress (Graham, 2022). Throughout the chapter, tools and micropractices guide implementation whether for personal or professional learning. The resource table in the chapter has links to several auditory or video opportunities emphasizing story. The following reflective practice guide is applied to the Lewis Blackman story (see Table 7.1) but can be applied to other stories as well.

MICROPRACTICES

MICROPRACTICE: STORY AS TEACHER

The Lewis Blackman story listed in Table 7.1 in Chapter 7 in the textbook provides a powerful tool to demonstrate the imperative of quality and safety competencies and interprofessional practice (American Association of Colleges of Nursing [AACN], 2021). Use the video in class with nursing, pharmacy, and medical students. The video can be paired with theory bursts on patient safety competencies, just culture, transparent communication, and interprofessional practice (see AACN Domains in Chapter 1). Use a reflective debriefing to help process the meaning of the story and identify lessons learned for behavior change. After their reflection, ask participants to write a 6-word story to illustrate what they learned about patient safety.

REFLECTIVE DEBRIEFING OF STORY:

1. What stands out in this situation?

   a. What is my immediate concern?

   _____

   _____

   b. Why do I think that?

   _____

   _____

2. What assumptions influence my thinking?

   a. What are potential biases?

   _____

   _____

   b. What could change my thinking?

   _____

   _____

3. What else could be going on?

   a. How can I be open to alternatives?

   _____

   _____

   b. What is the worst possibility?

   _____

   _____

4. What previous experiences may help?

    a. Have I seen this before?

        _____

        _____

    b. What is similar and different this time?

        _____

        _____

5. What are three takeaways from this story to inform my work?

    _____

    _____

6. Using the following guidelines, write a 6-word story based on your reflections from this story.

    _____

    _____

MICROPRACTICE: JOURNALING ABOUT COMMUNICATION: STORIES FROM MULTIPLE PERSPECTIVES

Write about an experience that has meaning for you, describing a time when you and another person communicated well (or didn't communicate well). Try to tell the story in as much detail as possible so that as you read it to others, they can see and hear the situation. It might be helpful to think about the following as you get started:

1. What was going on at the time? (Time of day, setting, individuals involved, etc.)

    _____

    _____

2. How did you know the communication was going well or not going well? What did you see or hear that told you this?

    _____

    _____

3. What were you concerned about at the time?

_____

_____

4. What was going through your head as the situation unfolded?

_____

_____

5. What were you feeling during and after the experience?

_____

_____

6. Did anything surprise you in the experience?

_____

_____

When you have finished writing your story, please write a second story from the perspective of another person who shared this same experience. Again, try to include as much detail as possible—and describe as clearly as you can what the situation looked like to that other person. What were that person's concerns? What do you suppose was running through their mind as the situation unfolded?

_____

_____

_____

_____

_____

_____

MICROPRACTICE: PROMPTS FOR LEARNING REFLECTION

1. One thing I learned today that I did not know before is . . .

_____

_____

2. One thing I knew before but now understand in a different way is . . .

_____

_____

3. I still have questions or concerns about . . .

_____

_____

MICROPRACTICE: THE 6-WORD AND 55-WORD STORY

Educators and facilitators can use a reflective writing technique based on two literary formats: the 6-word and 55-word story. Reflection rather than writing is the primary purpose. Reflecting helps choose words carefully to stay within six words. From the six words, participants expand their reflection to 55 words, remaining focused on clarity and message.

IMPLEMENTING THE 6-WORD REFLECTION:

- Make a list of three or four memorable experiences participants have participated in.

- Write the memories or experiences into a 6-word reflection (story).

- Choose words wisely, recognizing the power in words, and use only six.

- Focus on clarity and completeness to accurately encompass the impression of the event with a short phrase.

Examples of 6-word reflections:

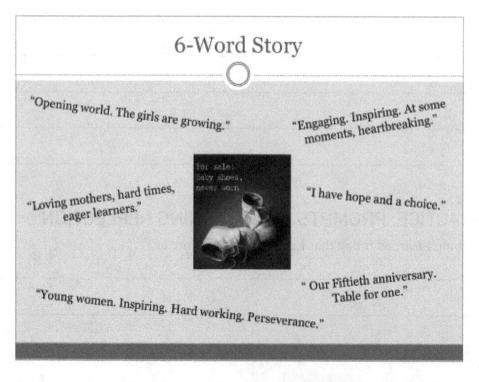

Write your 6-word story here: _____

EXPANDING TO THE 55-WORD STORY

After completing the 6-word reflection, continue reflecting to extend it into a *55-word story* to establish additional detail. The reflection must be exactly *55* words; it should tell a story and be reflective of the experience.

- Start by writing phrases, words, or important images.

- Edit once completed to trim to *55* words.

- Focus on clarity and the power of the words selected. Consider the narrative elements that make this story significant or special.

Examples of 55-word stories:

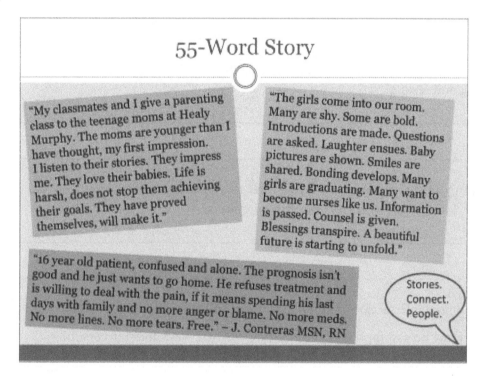

REFLECTIVE QUESTIONS

1. Why are stories considered a powerful learning tool?

_____

_____

2. We all have a story. Craft your story to share with someone by considering:

    a. What is a life-altering experience you have had that was a turning point?

    _____

    _____

    b. What values and intentions guided your actions?

    _____

    _____

    c. How have you responded to similar situations in light of this story?

    _____

    _____

3. Practice silence by remaining quiet for one minute. What did you hear? What were you thinking and feeling?

_____

_____

4. How can you cultivate active listening? Recall an incident today when you had to listen to another. How would you rate your listening skills?

_____

_____

5. Reflect on the intersection of story generation and the diagnostic process.

    a. How do assumptions influence how we first view another person?

    _____

    _____

    b. How can we as nurses hear the patient's full story to help the entire team in making care recommendations?

    _____

    _____

REFERENCES

Alteren, J. (2019). Narratives in student nurses' knowledge development: A hermeneutical research study. *Nurse Education Today, 76,* 51–55. https://doi.org/10.1016/j.nedt.2019.01.015

American Association of Colleges of Nursing. (2021). *The essentials: Core competencies for professional nursing education.* https://www.aacnnursing.org/Portals/42/AcademicNursing/pdf/Essentials-2021.pdf

Armstrong, G., Sherwood, G., Ironside, P., Cerbie Brown, E., & Wonder, A. (2022). Reflective practice: Using narrative pedagogy to foster quality and safety. In G. Sherwood & J. Barnsteiner (Eds.), *Quality and safety in nursing: A competency approach to improving outcomes,* 3rd ed. (pp. 301–320). Wiley.

Boykin, A., & Schoenhofer, S. O. (1991). Story as link between nursing practice, ontology, epistemology. *The Journal of Nursing Scholarship, 23*(4), 245–248. https://doi.org/10.1111/j.1547-5069.1991.tb00680.x

Caspersz, D., & Stasinska, A. (2015). Can we teach effective listening? An exploratory study. *Journal of University Teaching & Learning Practice, 12*(4). https://ro.uow.edu.au/jutlp/vol12/iss4/2

Charon, R. (2004). Narrative and medicine. *The New England Journal of Medicine, 350*(9), 862–864. https://doi.org/10.1056/NEJMp038249

Choperena, A., Oroviogoicoechea, C., Zaragoza Salcedo, A., Olza Moreno, I., & Jones, D. (2019). Nursing narratives and reflective practice: A theoretical review. *Journal of Advanced Nursing, 75*(8), 1637–1647. https://doi.org/10.1111/jan.13955

Graham, M. M. (2022). Navigating professional and personal knowing through reflective storytelling amidst Covid-19. *Journal of Holistic Nursing, 40*(4), 372–382. https://doi.org/10.1177/08980101211072289

Ironside, P. M., Brown, E. C., & Wonder, A. H. (2017). Narrative teaching strategies to foster quality and safety. In G. Sherwood & J. Barnsteiner (Eds.), *Quality and safety in nursing: A competency approach to improving outcomes,* 2nd ed. (pp. 221–232). Wiley-Blackwell.

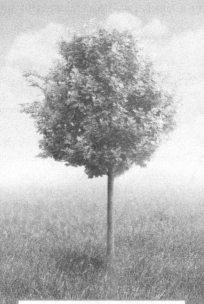

CHAPTER 8

REIMAGINING PRACTICING TOGETHER: REFLECTION IN SIMULATION-BASED LEARNING

Jennifer Alderman, PhD, RN, CNL, CNE, CHSE
Ashley A. Kellish, DNP, RN, CCNS, NEA-BC

LEARNING OBJECTIVES/SUBJECTIVES

- Describe application of simulation-based learning in nursing education and practice across the professional learning continuum.

- Distinguish types of reflective-practice theoretical models related to simulation learning.

- Determine best practices for simulation-based learning in interprofessional education.

- Delineate goals for a preferred future of simulation in nursing education and practice.

BEFORE YOU BEGIN

Learning for the real world of a practice-based discipline is complex. Multiple learning approaches are necessary to prepare novice nurses for the dynamics of working in any healthcare delivery setting. Learning is not only an academic responsibility; learning occurs across the professional life span. Nurse educators are emboldened to provide a transformative education for learners across the professional spectrum from prelicensure nursing education to continuing professional development in nursing practice.

Simulation-based learning grounded in adult learning and experiential learning theories is effective pedagogy for any stage of the nurse's career. Simulation learning is no longer an optional learning approach—it is a requirement for successful transition and competency development at any level of practice. Simulation-based learning is a method that provides a safe environment for optimal learning to occur. Robust, reflection-laden debriefs give learners the space needed to process their experiences and take concepts learned directly to patient care settings.

Simulation-based learning is founded on the principles of adult learning, experiential learning, and narrative pedagogy. Ignatian pedagogy provides a holistic model (see Figure 8.1) using five principal elements to guide learners and nurses in focusing on the larger picture and the needs of others (Moutin & Nowacek, 2012).

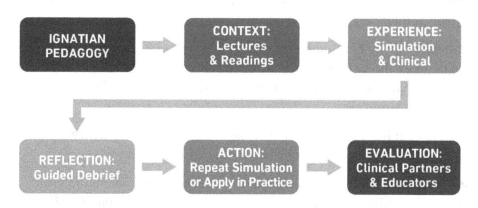

FIGURE 8.1   The five elements of Ignatian pedagogy.

The global pandemic led to reimagining the way nursing education is delivered in academic and practice settings. Answering the call created by the pandemic, educators pivoted to provide robust learning opportunities virtually and in-person. Taking a toll on the nursing workforce, the pandemic also created opportunities for innovation and forward-thinking on the part of educators and administrators alike. For an exhausted and, in some cases, decimated workforce, educators and administrators are creating meaningful learning experiences to prepare learners for practice, orient new nurses to practice, and provide continuing education for those who have been practicing.

The American Association of Colleges of Nursing (AACN, 2021) endorses simulation-based learning as a method by which competency-based education can be attained. Competency-based evaluation methods used in simulation-based learning need to include theoretical scaffolding approaches to evaluation, objective faculty assessments and learner self-assessments, and outcome evaluation based on knowledge and performance rather than relying on learner satisfaction and self-confidence (Cole, 2023; Rudolph et al., 2007).

Chapter 8 describes best practices in simulation-based learning in nursing education (INACSL Standards Committee et al., 2021) and practice including interprofessional education (Interprofessional Education Collaborative, 2016) and cites future directions expanding simulation in graduate nursing education (Hussein & Favell, 2022), telehealth (Cook, et al., 2022), virtual reality (Tolarba, 2021), and faculty orientation (Ross et al., 2022). The role of reflection as integral to simulation-based learning practice is based on reflection-before-action, reflection-in-action, reflection-on-action, and reflection-beyond-action (Alden & Durham, 2017). Applying the reflective practice model within simulation-based learning helps learners apply complex knowledge and encourages skill-based practice in achieving essential competencies.

MICROPRACTICES

Reflection and simulation-based learning form an ideal partnership working synergistically to maximize the effectiveness of the simulated practice experience. Reflection is important for planning and debriefing. Alden and Durham (2017) describe four reflective strategies for developing personal and professional learning goals to maximize learning opportunities and for translating to real-world practice: reflection-before-action, reflection-in-action, reflection-on-action, and reflection-beyond-action, presented in the following bullets.

- **Reflection-before-action:** Pre-simulation planning includes reflecting on knowledge, skills, attitudes, emotions, and past experiences. Important activities include orienting to the environment, explaining the process, discussing objectives of the activity, assigning roles, and presenting the simulation case.

- **Reflection-in-action:** Intra-simulation participants must think on their feet, huddle to problem solve, take team time outs to get on same page, or call for resources.

- **Reflection-on-action:** Debriefing is the guided reflection on individual and group performance, care of the patient, teamwork, communication, reactions, and decision-making led by trained facilitators and may include reviewing video recordings of the simulation itself.

- **Reflection-beyond-action:** Post-simulation reflection helps learners sustain what they learned for integrating into their work. One strategy is to have learners write a two-page debriefing paper describing challenges, application to practice, and questions that remain.

How would you use each of these reflective practices in planning a simulation-based learning activity?

_____

_____

_____

_____

MICROPRACTICE: REFLECTING WITH GOOD JUDGMENT

Quality and safety are essential competencies across all of nursing education, including learners, clinicians, and educators (AACN, 2021). To explore how reflective practice helps promote safety, engage in the following micropractice. This activity can occur in person or in the virtual environment (Rudolph et al., 2007).

Individually or in a group, describe a case scenario in which patient harm has occurred. Now, simulate a debriefing learning encounter by having participants engage in role-play of the scenario as interprofessional team members who were part of the event and now are debriefing. Each participant takes turns in playing different roles such as nurse, physician, educator, learner, or other team member. Work in pairs using an advocacy/inquiry approach to gain experiential learning of the difficult conversations occurring in the aftermath of preventable harms to patients.

Advocacy/inquiry questions may be based on the following questions (Rudolph et al., 2007):

- As a participant, how are you feeling after learning what happened in the scenario?

_____

_____

- Use the Plus/Delta Model to engage in what went well and what might be done differently next time.

    - What did you find of value in the scenario?

    _____

    _____

    - What could be improved next time?

    _____

    _____

- Conclude the debrief by summarizing major takeaways. For groups, ask the team to share one key learning point they have gained.

_____

_____

LEARNING NARRATIVE

The AACN has determined that the 21st-century nurse must practice as a skilled care coordinator across four spheres of care: disease prevention/promotion, chronic disease care, regenerative and restorative care, and hospice/palliative care while simultaneously maintaining safety and quality of care (AACN, 2021). Given these expectations, nurses are met with many competing priorities while providing patient-centered care. Prelicensure nurses frequently enter the workforce underprepared to face these pressures. Nurse educators are required to provide opportunities for prelicensure nurses to practice leadership skills such as effective communication, managing conflict, and increasing self-awareness. The purpose of the following leadership simulation was to improve the communication, conflict management, and self-awareness knowledge, skills, and attitudes of prelicensure nursing students (Alderman & Durham, 2022).

In collaboration with the university's Business School, the School of Nursing developed the *Peak Performance* leadership simulation to help prelicensure nursing students improve their leadership skills. During the simulation, the learner responds to a variety of patient care, team-based, and personal situations utilizing various means of communication such as emails, voice messages, and texts in the context of six patient care rounds. The learner must address as many scenarios per round as possible, being as efficient with time as possible. Small group debriefings were held in virtual breakout rooms. Students described their rationales for prioritizing and how they would handle conflicts they encountered. Students completed a reflection workbook after the debriefing and were offered the opportunity for one-on-one coaching sessions with the executive coaches from the Business School. Students completed pre/post assessments in which they evaluated their personal skills in self-awareness, communication, collaboration, openness, managing conflict, and managing others. The reflection workbook provided qualitative data related to self-evaluation of the following core values: empathy, integrity, and respect, along with a three-step action plan for improvement. Students noted improvement in knowledge and skills around communication and managing conflict, but they expressed frustration in the inability to complete all rounds of the simulation. Students were surprised by the complexity of care coordination awaiting them as they entered nursing practice.

Pre-licensure students increased their communication skills and obtained a better understanding of how to manage conflict in real-world circumstances fraught with competing priorities. Effective communication, conflict management, and self-awareness are critical to patient safety and providing quality care. Exposing students to the complex care coordination role of the nurse aligns well with the new AACN Essential Domains 2.9a–e and 5.2a–f (AACN, 2021).

The success of the nursing-focused Peak Performance simulation led educators to spread the model to an interprofessional version. Prelicensure nursing students, graduate nursing students, and medical students participated in a newly designed Peak Performance simulation focused on a discharge-planning case. The format was the same in that students received some introductory didactic information and then completed the simulation individually, answering reflection and prioritization questions. Business coaches led the debrief, and the simulation closed with a panel of interprofessional faculty discussing and reflecting on the challenges they faced when they transitioned to practice. All student participants completed pre/post surveys. Results showed significant gains in six leadership skills: self-awareness, communication, collaboration, openness, managing conflict, and managing others (Alderman & Durham, 2022).

The major points to take away here are:

- Nursing shifts are fraught with competing priorities amid complex care environments every day.

- Nurse educators are obligated to prepare nurses for complex care environments.

- Teamwork, communication, and conflict management are cornerstones of patient quality and safety.

- Providing high-quality leadership simulations with debriefing methods grounded in reflection led by skilled educators can improve the competencies of learners in the areas of teamwork, communication, conflict management, and self-reflection.

1. How have you handled competing priorities encountered in your nursing practice?

_____

_____

_____

2. After reflecting on your practice, what behaviors that you deem effective would you continue performing in your daily workflow and why?

_____

_____

_____

3. After reflecting on your practice, what behaviors would you stop doing?

_____

_____

_____

4. How has your thinking changed because of any insights you have obtained from this simulation?

_____

_____

_____

REFLECTIVE QUESTIONS

1. What shifts in the current healthcare environment are impacting nursing education and why?

_____

_____

_____

2. How does reflection improve nursing practice?

_____

_____

_____

3. How does interprofessional simulation impact the practice of healthcare professionals?

_____

_____

_____

4. What impact has the pandemic had on simulation-based learning?

_____

_____

_____

5. How would you reimagine new directions for simulation-based learning in nursing education and practice to capitalize on the innovative spirit resulting from the pandemic?

_____

_____

_____

REFERENCES

Alden, K., & Durham, C. (2017). Reflective practice in simulation-based learning. In S. Horton-Deutsch & G. Sherwood (Eds.), *Reflective practice: Transforming education and improving outcomes* (2nd ed., pp. 181–214). Sigma Theta Tau International.

American Association of Colleges of Nursing. (2021). *The essentials: Core competencies for professional nursing education.* https://www.aacnnursing.org/Portals/42/AcademicNursing/pdf/Essentials-2021.pdf

Cole, H. S. (2023). Competency-based evaluations in undergraduate nursing simulation: A state of the literature. *Clinical Simulation in Nursing, 76,* 1–16. https://doi.org/10.1016/j.ecns.2022.12.004

Cook, C., Becklenberg, A., Kendall, A., Leppke, A., & Vohra-Khulla, P. (2022). An interprofessional telehealth educational and simulation program for primary care student providers: A research pilot study. *Nursing Economics, 40*(5), 230–236.

Hussein, M. T. E., & Favell, D. (2022). Simulation-based learning in nurse practitioner program: A scoping review. *The Journal for Nurse Practitioners, 18*(8), 876–885. https://doi.org/10.1016/j.nurpra.2022.04.005

INACSL Standards Committee, Rossler, K., Molloy, M., Pastva, A, Brown, M., & Xavier, N. (2021, September). Healthcare simulation standards of best practice™ Simulation-enhanced interprofessional education. *Clinical Simulation in Nursing, 58,* 49–53. https://doi.org/10.1016/j.ecns.2021.08.015

Interprofessional Education Collaborative. (2016). *Core competencies for interprofessional collaborative practice: 2016 update.*

Mountin, S., & Nowacek, R. (2012). Reflection in action: A signature Ignatian pedagogy for the 21st century. In N. Chick, A. Haynie, & R. Gurung (Eds.), *Exploring more signature pedagogies: Approaches to teaching disciplinary habits of mind* (pp. 129–142). Stylus Publishing.

Ross, J. G., Dunker, K. S., Duprey, M. D., Parson, T., & Humphries, L. (2022). The use of simulation for clinical nursing faculty orientation: A multisite study. *Clinical Simulation in Nursing, 63,* 23–30. https://doi.org/10.1016/j.ecns.2021.11.001

Rudolph, J. W., Simon, R., Rivard, P., Dufresne, R. L., & Raemer, D. B. (2007). Debriefing with good judgment: Combining rigorous feedback with genuine inquiry. *Anesthesiology Clinics, 25*(2), 361–376. https://doi.org/10.1016/j.anclin.2007.03.007

Tolarba, J. E. L. (2021). Virtual simulation in nursing education: A systematic review. *International Journal of Nursing Education, 13*(3), 48–54. https://doi.org/10.37506/ijone.v13i3.16310

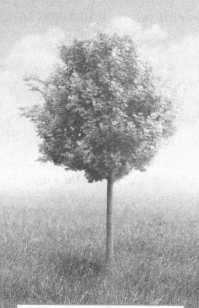

REFLECTIVE LEARNING: RECALIBRATING COLLABORATION AND EVALUATION FOR SAFETY AND QUALITY COMPETENCIES

Gail Armstrong, PhD, DNP, RN, ACNS-BC, CNE, FAAN
Gwen Sherwood, PhD, RN, FAAN, ANEF

LEARNING OBJECTIVES/SUBJECTIVES

- Apply various learning theories to nurses' professional development from academic learning across the professional life span.

- Describe reflective approaches reimagining ways to expand emotional intelligence and appreciative inquiry.

- Demonstrate reflective practices as a change model based on experiential learning, inquiry, and self-assessment for developing professional maturity.

- Examine reflective processes to make sense of contradictions in practice.

BEFORE YOU BEGIN

The centrality of reflective practice as a pivotal tenet of effective nursing education holds true for clinical nurses as well. Regardless of where one is on the professional journey, a practice of reflection strengthens a nurse's capacity for self-awareness, mindfulness, and situational awareness. Best developed in one's educational program, reflective practice is valuable to all nurses in a variety of clinical settings. Reflective practice means rethinking practice, one's relationships with others, and our feelings about performing certain tasks. Reflective practice is becoming more self-aware of one's own practice (Sherwood & Day, 2022).

This chapter applies various learning theories for co-creating reflective learning in interactive experiences to appreciate and develop ways to better understand nurses' work, explore and make sense of contradictions, and apply self-assessment to propel professional growth and development. Reflective practices that illustrate emotional intelligence (Horton-Deutsch & Sherwood, 2008) and appreciative inquiry (Merriel et al., 2022) guide deep reflections to analyze work experiences for developing tacit and other forms of knowledge. Examples showcase micropractices that educators and mentors can use to help learners and nurses develop reflective practice skills and explore how to integrate reflective approaches into learners' formative and summative clinical assessments and evaluative feedback (Armstrong et al., 2022).

Pairing reflective practice with standards of quality and safety facilitates an awareness of the disconnect that often accompanies a compromise to quality and safety (Day & Sherwood, 2022). In this disconnect lies the opportunity for understanding and improvement. Similar to nurse learners, nurse clinicians need time, space, and facilitation to debrief a safety event. Building intellectual muscle memory in reflective practice for nurse learners positions nurse clinicians to optimize the benefits of this essential skill set. Furthermore, evaluation modalities employed with nurse learners in educational programs are well-suited for the evaluation of vital aspects of the practice of nurse clinicians.

The chapter covers reflection as learning and reflection as assessment. Engaging learners in helping create reflective, learner-centered classroom and clinical environments, reflective course evaluation, and appreciative inquiry as a reflective change model instill habits of the mind that reinforce lifelong learning.

MICROPRACTICES

MICROPRACTICE: LEARNING FROM EXPERIENCE

It is said we do not learn from experience; we learn from reflecting on experience.

Reflective practice pedagogy, whether in academic or clinical settings, provides important opportunities for nurses to explore their professional and individual commitment to safe, quality care and their contribution to a positive work environment. Written reflective dialogue with teachers, mentors, or other nurses provides systematic learning; this reflection-on-action is a process of sense-making of experience, thus building tacit knowledge to move toward professional maturity.

Instilling a habit of reflection helps assure a growth mindset for continuous improvement personally and professionally. Reflecting daily on critical events helps make sense of contradictions, increases self-awareness, and leads to changes in work practices. A habit of the mind based on these four questions helps set a continuous learning approach.

Reflect on an event that has meaning for you:

* What went well?

_____

_____

* What can be improved?

_____

_____

* Considering this event, what was both satisfying and frustrating?

_____

_____

* What concerns do you still have?

_____

_____

MICROPRACTICE: WRITING PROMPTS FOR REFLECTION

Professionals must learn to communicate through writing, a learned skill. Reflection, however, is writing to learn. Guided prompts provide a more structured and meaningful approach to reflection. Start by maintaining a reflective journal using the following questions as initial prompts. The same questions can be used as discussion or writing prompts by educators, mentors, learners, and nurses for weekly writing assignments.

1. Describe your top three priorities for your nursing practice. What barriers are you encountering in achieving these priorities?

_____

_____

_____

2. Reflect on your most recent clinical experience. What caregiving challenges did you observe that impacted patient care quality and safety? Why do you say that?

_____

_____

_____

3. Describe a clinical experience that affirmed your decision to enter nursing.

_____

_____

_____

4. What was a notable experience from your time at work today? Why do you think it was important for you?

_____

_____

_____

5. When were you unsure of what to do today? How did you feel? What steps did you take to be able to make an informed decision?

_____

_____

_____

MICROPRACTICE: REFLECTING ON REFLECTING

Reflective practice touches our personal experiences and our beliefs and attitudes—and challenges our growth. As you complete micropractices within this guide, reflect on what you have learned, what has changed, and what questions remain.

1. From your reflections, what changes do you see in your perspectives about your work?

_____

_____

_____

2. What changes in your behavior indicate the benefits of reflection?

_____

_____

_____

3. Describe ways you have applied what you have learned from reflection to change your behaviors.

_____

_____

_____

4. What evidence in your reflections demonstrates your commitment to growing and changing through reflective practices?

_____

_____

_____

MICROPRACTICE: APPLYING REFLECTIVE LEARNING TO FEEDBACK

The dominant mode of instruction in nursing education (especially clinical education) has an expert-educator and novice-learner relationship. Changing the clinical learning paradigm to an open learning partnership aligned with transformative, interactive, experiential learning fits the goals and aims of reflection (Horsburgh & Ippolito, 2018). Engaging learners or nurses in reflective practice requires mutual openness to examine new ideas and the ability to listen and act appropriately; both learners and educators must adopt an open attitude. Innovative assessment strategies include narratives, unfolding cases, simulation, focus groups, rubrics, reflection-on-action, and appreciative inquiry.

Nurses do not learn from experience alone; deep learning comes from critically reflecting on experience. Bauer (2002) shared questions for evaluating learner participation in an online leadership course. Learners were given the following knowledge work questions for reflecting on their readings each week:

1. What concepts, theories, models, tools, techniques, and resources in the week's assigned readings did you find most valuable?

2. How might you use this information in your practice?

3. Why is the information important to your practice?

4. How will the knowledge improve your effectiveness as a clinician?

5. How does the knowledge and information help you understand the interdependence of system dynamics in terms of context, relationships, and trends?

6. Why care about the knowledge? How does it help you clarify values and manage professional purpose?

7. How does the knowledge gained advance your achievement of the nursing program outcomes and support your mastery of the essentials for preparation as a registered nurse?

8. What other thoughts, reflections, or significant learning have influenced your personal and/or professional development these past few weeks?

9. Create and pose a question of your own design to the members of your learning circle. Answer at least one question posed by a colleague in your learning circle.

Clark (2011) proposes a set of reflective questions for educators to ask in setting expectations for evaluation of reflective activities that can be used in didactic or clinical learning experiences:

1. Does the learner or nurse seek alternatives?

2. Does the learner or nurse view the experience from various perspectives?

3. Does the learner or nurse seek a framework, theoretical basis, or underlying rationale (of behaviors, methods, techniques, programs)?

4. Does the learner or nurse compare and contrast?

5. Does the learner or nurse put the experience into different or varied contexts?

6. Does the learner or nurse ask, "What if . . .?"

7. Does the learner or nurse consider consequences?

LEARNING NARRATIVE

Table 9.1 provides examples for learners and nurses in developing competencies defined both by QSEN skills and attitude elements, which are also exemplified in several domains from the 2021 AACN Essentials (adapted from Armstrong et al., 2017). Review the competency element in column two describing the competency in column one. Use the prompts in column three to reflect on your own practice, identify ways to improve, and consider additional learning needs.

TABLE 9.1	QUALITY AND SAFETY EDUCATION FOR NURSES' (QSEN) COMPETENCY ELEMENT AND AACN DOMAIN FOR CLINICAL REFLECTION PROMPTS	
QSEN AND AACN COMPETENCY	**COMPETENCY ELEMENT**	**PROMPT FOR CLINICAL REFLECTION**
Patient-Centered Care (AACN Domain 2: Person-Centered Care)	Value the patient's expertise with own health and symptoms (Attitude)	• What observable behaviors in your practice demonstrate this attitude? • How do you balance the need for efficiency in your practice and the time/space for this attitude and corresponding behaviors? • Are there clinical situations where this attitude is in conflict with another practice value?
	Value continuous improvement of own communication and conflict-resolution skills (Attitude)	• Consider nurses you have observed who role-model this attitude in their practice and describe what it looks like. • What are the difficult or uncomfortable aspects of this attitude? How does your own self-awareness help with the improvement process included in this attitude?
Teamwork and Collaboration (Domain 6: Interprofessional Education and Practice)	Demonstrate awareness of own strengths and limitations as a team member (Skills)	• How do clinicians demonstrate this skill? How would this look to their colleagues? • How does this skill facilitate healthy teamwork?
	Respect the unique attributes that members bring to a team, including variations in professional orientations and accountabilities (Attitude)	• How might you gain awareness of the varied professional approaches and accountabilities of colleagues on your healthcare team? Why is this important? • What examples have you observed of "respect" acted out on the healthcare team? How has this attitude enhanced team functioning (from a colleague perspective)? From a patient perspective?
Evidence-Based Practice (Domain 4: Scholarship for Nursing Practice)	Question rationale for routine approaches to care that result in less than desired outcomes or adverse events (Skills)	• This skill requires individuals or teams to speak up. What are your observations of an individual's or a team's comfort with speaking up to question rationale for routine approaches that are ineffective? • As a nursing leader, how can you impact the culture of a microsystem so that individuals and teams feel free to speak up about ineffective care?

Quality Improvement (Domain 5: Quality and Safety)	Appreciate that continuous quality improvement is an essential part of the daily work of all health professions (Attitude)	• How is this attitude promoted among nurse leaders? • What is your experience of the adoption of this attitude among all team members? • What are supporting and disabling factors for this attitude in the work processes or habits you have observed? How do you integrate this attitude as a core part of your nursing practice?

REFLECTIVE QUESTIONS

1. What do you value most about nurses' work? What do you value most about the contributions you make to nursing?

    _____

    _____

    _____

2. What are the core values and best practices evident/absent in the examples of the reflections shared in this chapter?

    _____

    _____

    _____

3. Describe three things that you commit to for improving patient safety What are the challenges and opportunities for achievement?

    a. _____

    _____

    b. _____

    _____

    c. _____

    _____

4. What are ways to integrate reflective practices more effectively into your teaching and/or learning in both didactic and workplace learning?

_____

_____

_____

REFERENCES

American Association of Colleges of Nursing. (2021). *The essentials: Core competencies for professional nursing education*. https://www.aacnnursing.org/Portals/42/AcademicNursing/pdf/Essentials-2021.pdf

Armstrong, G., Horton-Deutsch, S. & Sherwood, G. (2017). Reflection and mindful practice: A means to quality and safety. In S. Horton-Deutsch & G. Sherwood (Eds.), *Reflective practice: Transforming education and improving outcomes* (2nd ed., pp. 29–49). Sigma Theta Tau International.

Armstrong, G., Sherwood, G., Ironside, P., Cerbie Brown, E., & Wonder, A. (2022). Reflective practice: Using narrative pedagogy to foster quality and safety. In G. Sherwood & J. Barnsteiner (Eds.), *Quality and safety in nursing: A competency approach to improving outcomes* (3rd ed., pp. 301–320). Wiley-Blackwell.

Bauer, J. F. (2002). Assessing student work from chatrooms and bulletin boards. *New Directions for Teaching and Learning, 91,* 31–36.

Clark, D. R. (2011). *Learning through reflection*. www.nwlink.com/~donclark/hrd/development/reflection.html

Day, L., & Sherwood, G. (2022). Transforming education to transform practice: Using unfolding case studies to integrate quality and safety in subject-centered classrooms. In G. Sherwood & J. Barnsteiner (Eds.), *Quality and safety in nursing: A competency approach to improving outcomes* (3rd ed., pp. 268–300). Wiley-Blackwell.

Horsburgh, J., & Ippolito, K. (2018). A skill to be worked at: Using social learning theory to explore the process of learning from role models in clinical settings. *BMC Medical Education, 18*(1), 156. https://doi. org/10.1186/s12909-018-1251-x

Horton-Deutsch, S., & Sherwood, G. (2008). Reflection: An educational strategy to develop emotionally competent nurse leaders. *Journal of Nursing Management, 16*(8), 946–954. https://doi.org/10.1111/j.1365-2834.2008.00957.x

Merriel, A., Wilson, A., Decker, E., Hussein, J., Larkin, M., Barnard, K., O'Dair, M., Costello, A., Malata, A., & Coomarasamy, A. (2022). Systematic review and narrative synthesis of the impact of Appreciative Inquiry in healthcare. *BMJ Open Quality, 11*(2), e001911. https://doi.org/10.1136/bmjoq-2022-001911

Sherwood, G., & Day, L. (2022). Quality and safety in clinical learning environments. In G. Sherwood & J. Barnsteiner (Eds.), *Quality and safety in nursing: A competency approach to improving outcomes* (3rd ed., pp. 321–348). Wiley-Blackwell.

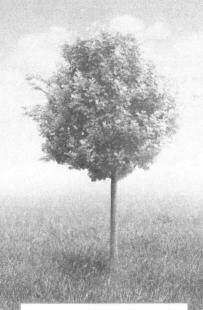

CHAPTER 10

RETHINKING HOW WE WORK TOGETHER: REFLECTIVE PRACTICES USING EMERGENT STRATEGY, LIBERATING STRUCTURES, AND CLEARNESS COMMITTEES

Sara Horton-Deutsch, PhD, RN, FAAN, ANEF, SGAHN
Gwen Sherwood, PhD, RN, FAAN, ANEF

LEARNING OBJECTIVES/SUBJECTIVES

- Identify the characteristics of effective and inclusive ways of working together in groups to help all belong.

- Describe theoretical frameworks that support reflective ways of working together.

- Discuss the value of reflection for creative problem-solving.

- Explore how emergent strategy, liberating structures, and clearness committees expand our capacity for creating more inclusive, engaging, adaptive, and resourceful learning and practice environments.

BEFORE YOU BEGIN

This chapter provides a comprehensive exploration of the importance of reflective practice, critical thinking, and Caring Science in group dynamics and interactions. The authors explore how entrenched behaviors, attitudes, and values can be reshaped through innovative reflective practices, creating inclusive environments where everyone belongs. They propose three processes (emergent strategy, liberating structures, and clearness committees) for engaging groups in identifying what is most important to chart a new path forward. These processes involve listening, creating authentic connections, providing support, and evolving to see possibility and wholeness. Educators are encouraged to explore the use of these three processes as active learning strategies to empower learners to take an active role in their education and to improve understanding, critical thinking skills, motivation, and preparation for real-world situations.

The chapter is grounded in several theoretical frameworks that emphasize the importance of self-reflection, critical thinking, and collaborative learning. These include Experiential Learning Theory, transformative learning theory, and complexity science.

Experiential Learning Theory (Kolb, 2014) emphasizes the importance of learning through direct experience, reflection, and application. In group settings, this framework involves engaging in activities that challenge assumptions, promote critical thinking, and facilitate self-reflection. *Transformative learning theory* views learning as a process of personal and social transformation that involves critically examining assumptions, beliefs, and values. From this perspective, group members engage in dialogue and activities that challenge assumptions and promote critical reflection on personal and societal values and beliefs.

Complexity science advocates for the importance of self-organization, adaptation, and emergence in complex systems. From this perspective, groups are viewed as complex adaptive systems that exhibit emergent behaviors that cannot be predicted by studying the behavior of individual members in isolation.

The chapter concludes by offering theory-based, practical, evidence-based ideas to reinvent group interactions regardless of size to enact reflective thinking. These ideas promote reflection-in-action and reflection-on-action. Principles from complexity science applied in emergent strategy, liberating structures, and clearness committees create more reflective, inclusive, and effective working environments.

In summary, the chapter encourages learners to embrace reflective practice, critical thinking, and Caring Science in their approach to group interactions and organizational relationships. It provides them with theoretical frameworks and practical strategies to navigate the complexities of these interactions and relationships and to foster a more collaborative, inclusive, and effective working environment.

MICROPRACTICES

MICROPRACTICE: EMERGENT STRATEGY

Emergent strategy is a concept in organizational theory that emphasizes the development of strategies through learning, adaptation, and continuous experimentation rather than relying solely on pre-determined, rigid plans. It recognizes that the healthcare environment is complex and uncertain; therefore, traditional top-down, long-term planning may not always be effective. For groups that are newly working together, social justice facilitator Adrienne Brown (2017) recommends setting some agreements in place. Reflect on the following agreements, and consider which ones would be useful in a group you have or are currently working with. Why do these micropractices matter?

- Listening from the inside out (a gut feeling matters)
- Engage tension; don't indulge in drama
- W.A.I.T.: Why am I talking?
- Make space, take space; balance speaking with listening
- Confidentiality
- Being open to learning
- Being open to someone else speaking your truth
- Building, not selling
- Yes/and, both/and
- Value the process as much as the outcome
- Assume the best intent
- Self-care and community care

MICROPRACTICE: LIBERATING STRUCTURES

Liberating structures are a collection of facilitation techniques and practices designed to involve everyone in a group and foster collaboration, creativity, and engagement. Developed by Lipmanowicz and McCandless (2013b), liberating structures aim to empower participants and break free from traditional hierarchical and top-down approaches to group interactions. The fundamental principle behind liberating structures is that every member of a group has valuable contributions to make, and by actively involving and engaging everyone, better decisions and outcomes can be achieved. These structures are simple and easy to learn; they can be used in various settings such as meetings, workshops, conferences, and team gatherings (Swenson et al., 2017). Figure 10.1 provides a list with short definitions of the liberating structure techniques to apply in your own group(s).

Liberating Structures Menu: Including and Unleashing Everyone   v 2.2

 Impromptu Networking
Rapidly share challenges and expectations, building new connections

 9 Whys
Make the purpose of your work together clear

 What, So What, Now What?
Together, look back on progress to-date and decide what adjustments are needed

 TRIZ
Stop counterproductive activities & behaviors to make space for innovation

 Appreciative Interviews
Discover & build on the root causes of success

 1-2-4-All
Engage everyone simultaneously in generating questions/ideas/suggestions

 User Experience Fishbowl
Share know-how gained from experience with a larger community

 15% Solutions
Discover & focus on what each person has the freedom and resources to do now

 25-To-10 Crowd Sourcing
Rapidly generate & sift a group's most powerful actionable ideas

 Troika Consulting
Get practical and imaginative help from colleagues immediately

 Conversation Café
Engage everyone in making sense of profound challenges

 Min Specs
Specify only the absolute "Must do's" & "Must not do's" for achieving a purpose

 Wise Crowds
Tap the wisdom of the whole group in rapid cycles

 Wicked Questions
Articulate the paradoxical challenges that a group must confront to succeed

 Drawing Together
Reveal insights & paths forward through non-verbal expression

 Improv Prototyping
Develop effective solutions to chronic challenges while having serious fun

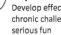 **Agreement-Certainty Matrix**
Sort challenges into simple, complicated, complex and chaotic domains

 Shift & Share
Spread good ideas and make informal connections with innovators

 Heard, Seen, Respected
Practice deeper listening and empathy with colleagues

 Social Network Webbing
Map informal connections & decide how to strengthen the network to achieve a purpose

 Design StoryBoards
Define step-by-step elements for bringing projects to productive endpoints

 Open Space
Liberate inherent action and leadership in large groups

 Discovery & Action Dialogue
Discover, spark & unleash local solutions to chronic problems

 Integrated~Autonomy
Move from either-or to robust both-and solutions

 Generative Relationships
Reveal relationship patterns that create surprising value or dysfunctions

 Critical Uncertainties
Develop strategies for operating in a range of plausible yet unpredictable futures

 Purpose-To-Practice
Define the five elements that are essential for a resilient & enduring initiative

 Ecocycle Planning
Analyze the full portfolio of activities & relationships to identify obstacles and opportunities for progress

 Panarchy
Understand how embedded systems interact, evolve, spread innovation, and transform

 What I Need From You
Surface essential needs across functions and accept or reject requests for support

 Celebrity Interview
Reconnect the experience of leaders and experts with people closest to the challenges at hand

 Helping Heuristics
Practice progressive methods for helping others, receiving help, and asking for help

 Simple Ethnography
Observe & record actual behavior of users in the field

FIGURE 10.1   Liberating structures menu.
Source: Lipmanowicz & McCandless, 2013a, p. 68

After reviewing the 33 structures, choose two that you haven't experienced before or find interesting.

1. How can you use one or both structures with a current group you are in?

_____

_____

_____

2. How might it/they increase collaboration? Creativity? Engagement? Reflecting on the liberating structures explored in the chapter (Conversation Cafes, 1-2-4-ALL, and TRIZ), how might they increase collaboration? Creativity? Engagement?

_____

_____

_____

LEARNING NARRATIVE

The COVID-19 pandemic has left an indelible mark on our global society. As educators regrouped to return to in-person classes, and workers in all settings dealt with the impacts on how they work, emotions rose to the surface. Using What/So What/Now What in our group, a liberating structure, provided a discussion platform to share experiences and move towards new beginnings. The guided reflective process provided a semi-structured way for everyone to share their responses in an inclusive, safe space free from judgment, and allowed diverse views to surface. By using appreciative constructive questions, the group remained focused on discussing how they wanted to reimagine the work environment and sustain positive changes that emerged from the pandemic. For the purposes here, you can follow the questions for your benefit by reflecting on your experience and the effect of the pandemic on your personal and professional life under number one and then reflect on the questions under numbers one and two as written. You can also try the exercise with your family, a group of peers, or with learners.

1. What: Understand the event.

    Reflect on the effects of the pandemic and identify the most striking impact on your personal and professional life. What stands out to you now? How is it still impacting your life?

_____

_____

_____

2. So what: Make sense of the facts and implications.

Reflecting on the points above, what were the things that surprised you the most?

- What are the most exciting things that were unavailable during the pandemic?

_____

_____

_____

- What were the most important strategies for your personal sustainment?

_____

_____

_____

- What strengths did you discover in yourself? In those around you?

_____

_____

_____

3. Now what: Set a course of action and new solutions.

- What was the most important gift of the pandemic that you continue to treasure?

_____

_____

_____

- What change are you committed to maintaining?

_____

_____

_____

• What is your preferred future going forward that the pandemic helped you redefine?

_____

_____

_____

REFLECTIVE QUESTIONS

1. What challenges and opportunities have you experienced working in nursing teams and interprofessional teams?

_____

_____

_____

2. How would you design a staff or faculty meeting using one of the strategies in the chapter?

_____

_____

_____

3. How do the theories presented help you to understand why the strategies are useful?

_____

_____

_____

4. Identify a critical question in your organization, and select one of the strategies from this chapter to organize for discussion.

Critical Question: _____

   a. Whom would you include?

_____

_____

    b. Where would you hold the session?

_____

_____

    c. How would you frame the question?

_____

_____

    d. What outcome do you hope for?

_____

_____

5. Compare and contrast the strategies described in this chapter with the usual problem-solving strategies.

_____

_____

_____

6. What are the strengths of the strategies described in this chapter?

_____

_____

_____

REFERENCES

Brown, A. M. (2017). *Emergent strategy: Shaping change, changing worlds.* AK Press.

Kolb, D. (2014). *Experiential learning: Experience as the source of learning and development.* Pearson FT Press.

Lipmanowicz, H., & McCandless, K. (2013a). *Liberating structures menu.* https://www.liberatingstructures.com/ls

Lipmanowicz, H., & McCandless, K. (2013b). *The surprising power of liberating structures: Simple rules to unleash a culture of innovation.* Liberating Structures Press.

Swenson, M., Sims, S., & McCandless, K. (2017). Reflective ways of working together: Using liberating structures. In S. Horton-Deutsch & G. Sherwood (Eds.), *Reflective practice: Transforming education and improving outcomes* (2nd ed., pp. 291–313). Sigma Theta Tau International.

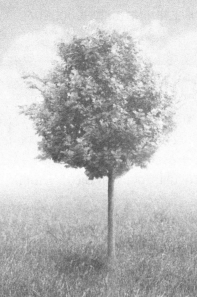

CHAPTER 11

PLURALISTIC POSSIBILITY: REFLECTIVE PRACTICES TO REFRAME OUR WORLD

Amber Young-Brice, PhD, RN, CNE
Melissa Shew, PhD
Jennifer Maney, PhD

LEARNING OBJECTIVES/SUBJECTIVES

- Connect AACN Essentials, guidelines, and competencies for nursing education to liberatory education and caring sciences in the service of caring for others.

- Interrogate shortcomings in "diversity of thought" as it currently tends to be used in organizations.

- Justify thinking in terms of pluralistic possibility as a strength in higher education, nursing practices, and leadership.

- Promote cross- and interdisciplinary expertise and leadership possibilities through pluralistic possibilities.

BEFORE YOU BEGIN

Chapter 11 introduces a theoretical and practical model called *pluralistic possibility* to help nurses, educators, and leaders address evolving needs beyond traditional notions of what we consider "diversity of thought." This chapter provides a comprehensive exploration of diversity of thought in the context of nursing, with a particular focus on the development of pluralistic possibilities in education, practice, and leadership.

The model of pluralistic possibility draws from liberatory education and consciousness-raising theories to challenge how we identify and transform problems. A significant part of the chapter is dedicated to language's role in discussing the concept of diversity of thought. Language evolves, and its meanings can be transferred from one realm of experience to another. The authors argue that cognitive diversity, or the inclusion of different ways of thinking and problem-solving, can enhance the effectiveness of healthcare teams. They caution, however, against using the concept of cognitive diversity or diversity of thought as a substitute for demographic diversity, arguing that both are important for creating inclusive and effective healthcare and educational environments. This transference of language between how we use "diversity" creates opportunities for interprofessional dialogue to identify and transform challenges to anticipate solutions and realities that are more future-directed and life-giving (Watson, 2017).

Reflective practices are woven throughout the chapter to help us transform our worldview and create possibilities for change. The authors emphasize the importance of self-awareness and empathy in nursing education and practice. They contend that these qualities and a commitment to equity and social justice are essential for providing effective and compassionate care. The authors highlight the role of education in fostering these qualities and promoting a culture of care that respects and values diversity. The JEDI (justice, equity, diversity, inclusion) model (Roy et al., 2022) is a reflective practice operationalizing equity and anti-oppression in nursing education.

The authors also discuss the concepts of gaslighting, ghosting, and breadcrumbing as forms of psychological manipulation that can occur in healthcare settings. They contend that understanding, naming, and addressing these newer concepts are crucial for creating the possibility to change them. We might say that naming these negative behaviors makes us more credible as knowers. This undermining of credibility might result in what philosopher Miranda Fricker (2007) calls "cognitive disablement," which "prevents [a person] from understanding a significant patch of her own experience: that is, a patch of experience which it is strongly in her interests to understand, for without that understanding she is left deeply troubled, confused, and isolated" (p. 151).

The chapter concludes with a call to action for nurses to develop self-awareness, empathy, and commitment to social justice. The authors provide reflective prompts to guide learners in developing their understanding of these concepts and applying them in their practice.

MICROPRACTICES

MICROPRACTICE: HOW DO STUDENTS WANT TO LEARN?

Operationalization of equity and anti-oppression in nursing education is outlined in the AACN Essentials, which threads justice, equity, diversity, and inclusion throughout the 10 domains (AACN, 2021; Roy et al., 2022). A school of nursing conducted a quality improvement project that integrated the concepts of justice, equity, diversity, and inclusion (JEDI) into their prelicensure nursing program. After conducting a needs assessment of what concepts students and faculty felt were missing in the curriculum related to JEDI, a curriculum revision was completed. Students responded positively about the incorporation of JEDI concepts, yielding the following themes (Roy et al., 2022):

1. Students had a greater awareness of the influence of social determinants of health.

2. Students appreciated the incorporation of different sexual orientations, genders, and ethnicities in case studies.

3. Students indicated the importance of correct pronoun use.

4. Students developed a better understanding of race, which is neither biological nor genetic.

5. Students were able to relate health disparities to social inequities rather than race.

Students suggested that faculty consider adding more JEDI concepts across the curriculum, including more examples of the assessment and care of BIPOC individuals, and that different disease manifestations be included (Roy et al., 2022).

A recent student survey, Student Voice Pulse Survey of $N = 1,250$ undergraduate students, revealed that students learn best through use of case studies (learning narratives) and discussions (Flaherty, 2023).

REFLECTIVE QUESTION

How can you infuse JEDI concepts through a pluralistic lens in a manner consistent with what students are indicating they learn best?

_____

_____

In any model of education, we must be vigilant about how people in relative positions of power—educators, practitioners, and leaders of any kind—should aim to cultivate personal self-awareness. A lack of self-awareness can translate to superficial empathy in line with expectations of professionalism, rather than nurtured through awareness of the complex lives of our students, patients, and colleagues (Wong et al., 2021). Further, the current focus on evidence-based practice (versus a more caring approach of evidence-informed practice), outcomes, and standards de-emphasize human relationships, empathy, and compassion (Eckroth-Bucher, 2010; Ghouse, 2022).

REFLECTIVE QUESTIONS

1. What are ways we can build a capacity for empathy through critical self-reflection and introspection?

   _____

   _____

2. How can we become conscious and break our biases toward fellow humans?

   _____

   _____

MICROPRACTICE: DEVELOPING EMPATHY

Empathy in education and clinical practice stems from the development of a holistic, empathic practice (McKinnon, 2018). Fostering a holistic empathic practice means embodying the process of empathy and not merely using it in isolation (McKinnon, 2018).

McKinnon (2018) outlines the antecedents of empathy:

1. Engagement
2. Listening and "echoing"
3. An informed awareness of another's circumstances (cognitive empathy)
4. A good imagination
5. Relating the product of that imagination to the self (affective empathy)

REFLECTIVE QUESTIONS

Reflect on the antecedents that you readily possess and those where you have room for growth. Now, consider the following reflective questions as a guide to fostering a holistic empathic practice.

1. How can you foster these elements in your classroom or practice setting?

   _____

   _____

   _____

2. How can you develop imagination, which McKinnon indicates is at the heart of empathy, as a way of being?

_____

_____

_____

LEARNING NARRATIVE

In nursing practice, even while a nursing student, compassion and self-awareness are essential to well-being and the ability to interact with and provide care for others. Developing compassion and self-awareness requires ongoing intentional practices. According to Younas and Rasheed, "Becoming self-aware requires continuous reflection and learning about self in different situations" (2018, p. 222). Consider the following reflective framework by Becker-Phelps (2023) that encourages the development of self-awareness through STEAM and how this framework could fit personally or professionally in a classroom or practice setting:

- **S-Sensations**

  What do I sense in my body? Think about a scenario or situation you've faced or anticipate facing in school or practice. How does your body feel when you think about this situation? Take a mindful approach and scan your body from your head to your toes.

- **T-Thoughts**

  What am I thinking? When you think about the scenario or situation, what sort of thoughts are you having? Are they self-critical thoughts including "should"? If you are having trouble thinking about your thoughts, try journaling or sharing with a trusted friend or colleague.

- **E-Emotions**

  What am I feeling? This is where you lean into what you're feeling when thinking about the scenario or situation. Self-critical thoughts can cause negative consequences and subsequent emotions that lead to stress, exhaustion, and possibly powerlessness (Younas & Rasheed, 2018).

- **A-Actions**

  How have I been acting/reacting? Pay attention to the impact of your thoughts and feelings and what sort of behaviors this situation has elicited. Negative thoughts and emotions can lead to drastic actions, whereas compassionate self-awareness of the thoughts and emotions can help you discern how to rationally navigate the situation.

- **M-Mentalizing**

  "Do I really get what's going on for me and understand what is motivating my actions?" Or "Do I really get what's going on for the other person and understand what is motivating their actions?" This aspect of the STEAM framework helps us get towards pluralistic possibility by considering ourselves but also others in this self-awareness process.

REFLECTIVE QUESTION

How can you incorporate creating self-awareness through STEAM to build your empathy skills?

_____

_____

_____

REFLECTIVE QUESTIONS

If no one person or disciplinary expertise is likely to completely solve in a lasting way a truly pressing problem, the task becomes how we might honor the expertise around us to identify, transform, and solve problems not only on a large scale but also in daily experiences in our classrooms, institutions, and organizations.

1. What other types of societal issues or concerns could be tackled by this approach?

_____

_____

_____

2. Which disciplines could begin to address these issues in your context?

_____

_____

_____

3. What are some specific collaborative strategies (or pluralistic possibilities) that could move these issues forward in meaningful ways?

_____

_____

_____

4. Is diversity of thought enough to get individuals to consider systemic inequities in their settings, or is something more needed to serve populations in a just way? Why or why not?

_____

_____

_____

5. How might the language in nursing education or healthcare settings evolve to best reflect all peoples' lived experiences?

_____

_____

_____

6. How does the evolution of language impact our perspectives on caring for others?

_____

_____

_____

REFERENCES

American Association of Colleges of Nursing. (2021). *The essentials: Core competencies for professional nursing education.* https://www.aacnnursing.org/Portals/42/AcademicNursing/pdf/Essentials-2021.pdf

Becker-Phelps, L. (2023). *Gain self-awareness through STEAM. Compassionate self-awareness.* http://drbecker-phelps.com/home/wp-content/uploads/2019/09/STEAM.pdf

Eckroth-Bucher, M. (2010). Self-awareness. A review and analysis of a basic nursing concept. *Advances in Nursing Science, 33*(4), 297–309. https://doi.org/10.1097/ANS.0b013e3181fb2e4c

Flaherty, C. (2023) Survey: Students cite barriers to success, seek flexibility. *Inside Higher Ed.* https://www. insidehighered. com/news/2023/02/14/survey-top-five-barriers-student-success

Fricker, M. (2007). *Epistemic injustice: Power and the ethics of knowing.* Oxford University Press. https://doi.org/10.1093/acprof:oso/9780198237907.001.0001

Ghouse, M. M. (2022). Shaping pluralistic cohesive societies. *Academicus International Scientific Journal, 13*(26), 154–160. https://doi.org/10.7336/academicus.2022.26.10

McKinnon, J. (2018). In their shoes: An ontological perspective on empathy in nursing practice. *Journal of Clinical Nursing, 27*(21-22), 3882–3893. https://doi.org/10.1111/jocn.14610

Roy, K., Hunt, K., Sakai, K., & Fletcher, K. (2022). Social justice in nursing education: A way forward. *Journal of Nursing Education, 61*(8), 447–454. https://doi.org/10.3928/01484834-20220602-05

Watson, J. (2017). Global advances in human caring literacy. In S. Lee, P. Palmieri, & J. Watson (Eds.), *Global advances in human caring literacy* (pp. 3–12). Springer.

Wong, S. H. M., Gishen, F., & Lokugamage, A. U. (2021). Decolonizing the medical curriculum: Humanizing medicine through epistemic pluralism, cultural safety, and critical consciousness. *London Review of Education, 19*(1), 1–22. https://doi.org/10.14324/LRE.19.1.16

Younas, A., & Rasheed, S. P. (2018). Compassionate self-awareness: A hidden resource for nurses for developing a relationship with self and patients. *Creative Nursing, 24*(4), 220–224. https://journals.sagepub.com/doi/abs/10.1891/1078-4535.24.4.220

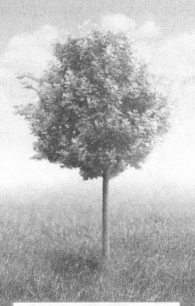

CHAPTER 12

REDESIGNING ACADEMIC AND PRACTICE PARTNERSHIPS: REFLECTIVE COMMUNITIES THAT LEARN AND PRACTICE TOGETHER

Eileen Fry-Bowers, PhD, JD, RN, CPNP-PC, FAAN

LEARNING OBJECTIVES/SUBJECTIVES

- Examine theoretical frameworks and models defining "reflective learning community."

- Differentiate between an academic-practice partnership created for the purpose of developing a clinical placement agreement versus one created for the purpose of reflective learning.

- Discuss the attributes needed for a successful academic-practice partnership to function as a reflective learning community.

- Describe how reflective academic-practice partnerships support the implementation of guidelines and competencies for nursing education.

- Explore the role of design thinking in creating a well-functioning academic-practice reflective learning community benefiting learners, educators, and clinicians.

BEFORE YOU BEGIN

Merriam-Webster defines *partnership* as "a relationship resembling a legal partnership and usually involving close cooperation between parties having specified and joint rights and responsibilities" (Merriam-Webster, 2023). Under this definition, most schools and programs of nursing and most healthcare entities may have hundreds of partnerships. Certainly, the nursing faculty shortage and increasingly limited supply of clinical sites available for learning experiences incentivize academic and practice entities to forge relationships that meet each institution's needs, often formalized through "clinical affiliation agreements" or "memoranda of understanding." Even so, many of these relationships do not create or facilitate conditions that foster the actualization of the goals stated in the AACN Academic Nursing (2016) Manatt Health Report.

Chapter 12 explores the historical evolution of nursing education as a practice-based discipline and the necessity of integrating didactic and practice-based learning and proposes co-creating alternative solutions. Reflections using hindsight, insight, and foresight perspectives (Pesut, 2019) examine the evolution of academia's relationships with healthcare delivery systems and its reliance on workplace learning in preparing nursing's workforce. Foresight reenvisions academic-practice partnerships as reflective learning communities that can learn and grow together.

Professional learning communities provide a structured space for people to connect, collaborate, and align around shared aspirational and practical goals and work across boundaries while holding members accountable to a common agenda, values, metrics, processes, and outcomes. Participants share and reflect on experiences and learn from each other, deepening collective knowledge and thereby improving their ability to achieve goals, make change, and potentially transform their industries. Learning communities provide a mechanism for connecting organizations, agencies, and philanthropies to engage in collective inquiry and action and promote scaling of promising practices (Stoll et al., 2006).

The rapid pace of change in society, and healthcare specifically, requires that learners be prepared to work in evolving systems that promote human well-being and resilience. Designing appropriately resourced, practical educational processes that benefit learners, the health system, and society requires frank discussions about deeply challenging issues. These conversations can only take place where there is an alignment about what is important, what is a priority, and what is valued within organizations, a commitment of time, empathy for the demands placed on each institution, and aligning incentives driving decisions within organizations. As a reflective learning community, academia and practice settings can co-design learning processes; they each inform the other through collaborative inquiry, reflective learning, and deliberative action in a continuous, collaborative, inclusive, learning-oriented, growth-promoting manner.

MICROPRACTICES

Nursing education institutions and nursing practice systems partnerships are essential for preparing the future nursing workforce. The following micropractices guide discussion for how these partnerships can join together to create a reflective learning community.

MICROPRACTICE: HINDSIGHT, INSIGHT, AND FORESIGHT

A reflective model of hindsight, insight, and foresight is a useful micropractice to examine organizations and systems to review the larger picture and assess directions for the future.

Identify at least one of the academic practice partnerships your organization is involved in:

_____

- **Hindsight:** Looking back for lessons learned

  - What are historical factors that have impacted how the partnership is formulated, goals, operations, and outcomes?

  _____

  _____

- **Insight:** Lessons learned applied in current situations

  - What are current healthcare delivery trends and practices impacting the relationship between academic and practice partners?

  _____

  _____

- **Foresight:** Looking towards the future

  - What are the primary goals and aims of the partnership? How can each partner contribute in a collaborative manner?

  _____

  _____

LEARNING NARRATIVE

Designing a reflective learning community requires an intentional commitment to creating a shared space to promote connection, collaboration, and clear communication. Partners in the community must be willing to continuously examine their individual and collective efforts, which requires trust, respect, and sharing of common values and goals.

A large public safety-net metropolitan health system has served as a clinical practice site for a private school of nursing for more than 20 years. The director of the prelicensure nursing program regularly communicates with the health system's director of professional education to arrange clinical experiences for learners. While cordial and professional, their relationship exists only to support this clinical placement function. They have no other regular interaction. Several nurses in the health system serve as adjunct clinical instructors for the school's nursing programs, and many direct care nurses routinely precept learners during their clinical experiences. Each entity faces significant challenges brought on by the rapid pace of change in the healthcare industry and higher education. The chief nursing officer of the health system and the dean of the school of nursing believe that each organization has much to offer the other organization, and they wish to form a partnership that will enable both entities to thrive in the future. They hope to design a reflective learning community that learns and practices together.

1. What should the leaders consider as they begin to form this academic-practice partnership?

_____

_____

_____

2. What questions should they be asking? And of whom?

_____

_____

_____

3. What organizational characteristics require consideration?

_____

_____

_____

4. Who are the community partners, and what role will they play in this partnership?

_____

_____

_____

5. What resources are available to them as they design this learning community?

_____

_____

_____

6. How will the leaders and interested participants measure the success of this effort?

_____

_____

_____

REFLECTIVE QUESTIONS

1. How can the theoretical frameworks and models explored in this chapter guide the development of a reflective learning community for enhancing collaboration and building evolutionary learning relationships?

_____

_____

_____

2. What are some key differences between a partnership focused on developing a clinical placement agreement and one focused on creating a reflective learning environment? How can these differences impact the overall goals and outcomes of the partnership for all involved?

_____

_____

_____

3. What personal attributes do you think are essential for creating a successful reflective learning community? In what ways can you cultivate these attributes within yourself and collaborate with others involved to foster a supportive and effective academic-practice partnership?

_____

_____

_____

4. How can reflective academic-practice partnerships support the implementation of guidelines and competencies for nursing education?

_____

_____

_____

5. What specific strategies promote collaboration, shared learning, and continuous improvement of nursing education within the context of academic-practice partnerships?

_____

_____

_____

REFERENCES

American Association of Colleges of Nursing. (2016). _Advancing healthcare transformation: A new era for academic nursing._ https://www.aacnnursing.org/Portals/0/PDFs/Publications/AACN-New-Era-Report

American Association of Colleges of Nursing. (2021). _The essentials: Core competencies for professional nursing education._ https://www.aacnnursing.org/Portals/42/AcademicNursing/pdf/Essentials-2021.pdf

Merriam-Webster. (2023). Partnership. In _Merriam-Webster online dictionary._ https://www.merriam-webster.com/dictionary/partnership?utm_campaign=sd&utm_medium=serp&utm_source=jsonld

Pesut, D. J. (2019). Anticipating disruptive innovations with foresight leadership. _Nursing Administration Quarterly, 43_(3), 196–204. https://doi.org/10.1097/NAQ.0000000000000349

Stoll, L., Bolam, R., McMahon, A., Wallace, M., & Thomas, S. (2006). Professional learning communities: A review of the literature. _Journal of Education Change, 7_(4), 221–258. https://doi.org/10.1007/s10833-006-0001-8

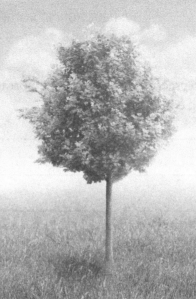

THE VALUE OF EMANCIPATORY NURSING PRAXIS AND CARING SCIENCE IN AN ERA OF LEGISLATIVE CENSORSHIP

Robin R. Walter, PhD, RN, CNE

LEARNING OBJECTIVES/SUBJECTIVES

- Analyze the implications of the current sociopolitical climate towards social justice, diversity, equity, and inclusion in higher education in general and nursing education specifically.

- Describe the learning process nurses experience in becoming social justice allies and equity advocates.

- Explain how a relational emancipatory pedagogy, grounded in Caring Science, can be used to educate nurses as social justice allies and equity advocates.

- Reflect on how social identity impacts nurse engagement with clients, coworkers, and peers.

BEFORE YOU BEGIN

Chapter 13 delves into the themes of reflective practice, critical thinking, and Caring Science through the implementation of relational emancipatory pedagogy and emancipatory nursing praxis. The chapter emphasizes the importance of educating nurses as equity advocates and social justice allies, and it provides a road map for achieving this goal despite current political and legislative challenges.

The author argues that social justice, diversity, equity, and inclusion teachings should be firmly grounded in nursing science, pedagogy, and learning processes. The chapter introduces the concepts of Caring Science, relational emancipatory pedagogy, and emancipatory nursing praxis as ways to move forward when the values held sacred in the nursing profession are being legislatively censored across the nation (Lu et al., 2023). In addition to the social justice issues identified in the chapter, facilitators may want to broaden the potential discussion topics to include Szulecki's (2023) top social justice stories of 2022. Weitzel et al. (2020) also provide examples of resistance movements and how nurses become allies with racially marginalized and oppressed populations.

The chapter discusses the concept of privilege and its intersection with oppression, creating complex social identities for each individual. The author encourages readers to reflect on their social identity and how it may prepare them to become allies. The chapter also addresses common objections and rebuttals that individuals in the early stages of learning about social justice may have, providing a platform for critical, reflective, and collaborative discussions. Facilitators are encouraged to read the final chapter in DiAngelo (2017), as the author offers guidance on ways to reframe and reflect on the questions posed in the learning narrative.

The chapter concludes with a call to action for nurses to become social justice allies, a process described as a lifelong journey of authentic collaboration of the "privileged" with the "other," with the ultimate goal of emancipation for both.

KEY CHAPTER THEMES

1. Diversity, equity, and inclusion education censored by state legislatures.

2. Aligning Caring Science philosophy, relational emancipatory pedagogy, and the theory of emancipatory nursing praxis in learning to become equity advocates/social justice allies in nursing.

3. The role of individual and social group identity in recognizing and addressing unearned privilege, structural power, and systemic oppression.

4. The challenges of—and absolute necessity for—critical self-reflection of personal socialization processes that create and sustain unconscious bias toward specific populations.

MICROPRACTICES

Engaging in micropractices related to social justice issues can help develop the stamina to become a social justice ally. These practices encourage self-awareness, critical thinking, and a commitment to positive change. Here are some reflective practices that nurses can incorporate into their journey toward becoming social justice allies.

MICROPRACTICE: SELF-EXAMINATION OF BELIEFS AND BIASES

Reflect on your beliefs, values, and biases related to social justice issues. Consider how your upbringing, education, and experiences have shaped your perspective.

Ask yourself challenging questions like:

1. What stereotypes or prejudices do I hold?

_____

_____

2. How do my privileges (e.g., race, gender, socioeconomic status) influence my worldview?

_____

_____

3. Am I open to reevaluating my beliefs?

_____

_____

MICROPRACTICE: ACTIVE LISTENING AND EMPATHY

Practice active listening when engaging in conversations with individuals from diverse backgrounds. Seek to understand their experiences and perspectives without judgment.

Develop empathy by putting yourself in others' shoes. Reflect on how you would feel in similar situations and how systemic injustices might affect you personally.

MICROPRACTICE: CONTINUOUS LEARNING

Engage in ongoing education about social justice issues. Attend workshops and lectures on racial justice, gender equity, LGBTQ+ rights, and more.

Read books, articles, and research papers written by scholars and activists in social justice. Consider joining or forming reading groups to discuss these materials.

MICROPRACTICE: CRITICAL REFLECTION ON MEDIA AND CULTURE

Analyze your media, including movies, TV shows, news sources, and social media. Reflect on how they portray different groups and issues.

Question the narratives presented in media, and consider their potential impact on society's perceptions and biases.

MICROPRACTICE: ENGAGEMENT IN CRITICAL DIALOGUE

Actively participate in discussions, debates, and dialogues about social justice issues. Encourage respectful and open conversations within your academic and social communities.

Reflect on the impact of your words and actions on others during these discussions. Strive to create a safe and inclusive space for diverse voices.

MICROPRACTICE: COMMUNITY INVOLVEMENT

Reflect on your role within your college community and the broader society. Consider how you can contribute to social justice through volunteering, advocacy, or activism.

Engage in service-learning experiences that allow you to work directly with marginalized communities and reflect on the lessons learned from these experiences.

MICROPRACTICE: SELF-CARE AND RESILIENCE

Recognize that engaging in social justice work can be emotionally challenging. Reflect on the importance of self-care and resilience-building to sustain your commitment to allyship.

Develop strategies for managing stress, anxiety, and burnout while continuing to advocate for social justice.

MICROPRACTICE: FEEDBACK AND ACCOUNTABILITY

Be open to receiving feedback from peers and mentors regarding your allyship efforts. Reflect on how you can use constructive criticism to improve your advocacy.

Hold yourself accountable for your actions and commitments. Reflect on instances where you may have fallen short and use them as opportunities for growth.

REFLECTIVE QUESTION

Has someone recently questioned your allyship or suggested you should perform it in a different manner? If so, how can you improve?

_____

_____

_____

Reflective practice is a key component of personal and social transformation. Nurses who engage in these reflective micropractices can develop a deeper understanding of social justice issues and actively contribute to positive change in their communities and beyond.

LEARNING NARRATIVE

The primary goal of this chapter is to demonstrate the science, pedagogy, and learning processes educators can use in teaching nurses to become social justice allies. Raising awareness and deepening students' consciousness of social justice, diversity, and equity will inevitably engage ideas and experiences new to many students that may be difficult to understand. There will be rebuttals and objections to some of these ideas by educators and students alike. Many of these objections, however, are predictable.

This learning activity asks you to critically, reflectively, and collaboratively wrestle with possible answers to the following rebuttals commonly offered by individuals who are in the early stages of learning about social justice (adapted from DiAngelo, 2017). Your goal is to develop thoughtful responses that promote understanding and awareness among individuals in the early stages of learning about social justice. You are encouraged to draw upon the concepts and strategies discussed in the chapter on teaching nurses to become social justice allies. Consider how to effectively address these objections while fostering empathy, critical thinking, and a commitment to social justice.

CITING EXCEPTIONS TO THE RULE

- "Barack Obama was elected President, so racism has ended in the US."
- "I have a friend who is Latina, and she is the CEO of the company."
- "My professor is openly gay, and he still got tenure."

Reply to one of the above objectives by using strategies from this chapter. Strive for an effective response that fosters empathy, critical thinking, and a commitment to social justice.

_____

_____

APPEALING TO A UNIVERSALIZED HUMANITY

- "Why can't we all just be humans?"

- "We all bleed red."

- "It's focusing on our differences that divides us."

Reply to one of the above objectives by using strategies from this chapter. Strive for an effective response that fosters empathy, critical thinking, and a commitment to social justice.

_____

_____

INSISTING ON IMMUNITY FROM CULTURAL SOCIALIZATION

- "I was taught to see everybody the same."

- "My parents raised me to be colorblind."

- "My parents told me that it didn't matter that I was a girl. I could be anything I wanted."

- "That's not my experience."

Reply to one of the above objectives by using strategies from this chapter. Strive for an effective response that fosters empathy, critical thinking, and a commitment to social justice.

_____

_____

IGNORING INTERSECTIONALITY

- "I'm oppressed as a lesbian, so I might be white, but I have no privilege."

- "I think the true oppression is poverty. If we address that, then the other oppressions will disappear."

Reply to one of the above objectives by using strategies from this chapter. Strive for an effective response that fosters empathy, critical thinking, and a commitment to social justice.

_____

_____

REFUSING TO RECOGNIZE STRUCTURAL AND INSTITUTIONAL POWER

- "Women are just as sexist as men."

- "People of color are racist too."

Reply to one of the above objectives by using strategies from this chapter. Strive for an effective response that fosters empathy, critical thinking, and a commitment to social justice.

_____

_____

REFLECTIVE QUESTIONS

1. What are my individual and social group identities, and how does that affect my current life experiences?

_____

_____

_____

2. What are my own personal biases about others, and how can I be prepared to monitor, address, and/or manage these biases?

_____

_____

_____

3. How can I make the unconscious things I have been socialized to believe more conscious so that I can wrestle with them?

_____

_____

_____

4. How can I understand that being more aware of what I have been socialized to believe, no matter how embarrassing and shameful those beliefs are, is liberating for the oppressed and the privileged?

_____

_____

_____

5. What does it mean to be a social justice ally? How can I work systemically to foster more justice and equity? How can I advocate for social justice, identifying ways to create change and promote social justice in our communities and the greater society?

_____

_____

_____

6. How do systems of oppression function in society, and how is that system maintained and perpetuated? How does this play out on individual, institutional, and societal levels? How does this play out consciously/intentionally and unconsciously/unintentionally?

_____

_____

_____

7. Reflect on your practice setting.

   a. Who is not being heard or represented?

   _____

   _____

   b. How does your reflection on your own privilege and oppression inform a new way of seeing this situation?

   _____

   _____

REFERENCES

DiAngelo, R. (2017). *Is everyone really equal? An introduction to key concepts in social justice education* (2nd ed.). Teachers College Press.

Lu, A., Elias, J., June, A. W., Charles, J. B., Marijolovic, K., Roberts-Grmela, J., & Surovell, E. (2023, May 15). DEI legislation tracker. *The Chronicle of Higher Education*. https://www.chronicle.com/article/here-are-the-states-where-lawmakers-are-seeking-to-ban-colleges-dei-efforts

Szulecki, S. (2023). The top social justice stories of 2022. *American Journal of Nursing, 123*(1), 14–15.

Weitzel, J., Wesp, l., Graf, M., Dressel, A., Mkandawire-Valmu, L. (2020). The role of nurses as allies against racism and discrimination: An analysis of key resistance movements of our time. *Advances in Nursing Science, 43*(2), 102–113.

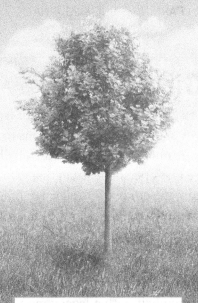

CHAPTER 14

REIMAGINING LEADERSHIP: A LEGACY PERSPECTIVE

Daniel J. Pesut, PhD, RN, FAAN

LEARNING OBJECTIVES/SUBJECTIVES

- Define the concept of legacy leadership to inform personal and professional reflection about career contributions to nursing education, practice, research, and policy.

- Describe five practices of legacy leadership to gain insight into ways of leading, being, and doing to activate a legacy leadership plan.

- Appreciate the role of personal strengths, values, and contribution appraisals to gain insights about one's vision, mission, and legacy.

- Determine a legacy through reflection-in and -on legacy leadership principles and practices.

- Reimagine one's professional nursing journey to enact legacy leadership principles and practices.

BEFORE YOU BEGIN

Chapter 14 describes and discusses principles and practices of legacy leadership for guiding personal and professional reflection on one's legacy contributions to nursing education, practice, research, and policy. Reflecting on one's purpose, values, and contributions to the profession promotes self-knowledge to maximize one's personal strengths, values, and contributions. The principles of legacy leadership fit within the context of reflective practice and Caritas Processes that are integrated throughout this book (Pesut, 2019). A series of micropractices to discern personal strengths, values, and contributions help in reimagining leadership with legacy perspectives. The author's personal reflections and learning narrative are a key feature of the chapter, with reflective questions to promote learning and reflection for one's own leadership journey.

Legacies can be planned and made explicit with a legacy map. *Legacy planning* is an interactive process that integrates aspects of career goal planning, attends to issues of meaning and purpose in terms of self and others, and is a shared experience between mentors and mentees as well as between leaders and followers.

Kouzes and Posner (2006, p. 180) write, "Legacies are not the result of wishful thinking. They are the results of determined doing. The legacy you leave is the life you lead. We live our lives daily. We leave our legacy daily. The people you see, the decisions you make, and the actions you take—they are what tell your story." Sandstrom and Smith (2017) note that legacy leadership is not what you leave behind; it is how you influence others to accomplish change.

The chapter details the be-attitudes of legacy leadership: vision and values, collaboration and innovation, influence and inspiration, difference and community, and responsibility and accountability (Sandstrom & Smith, 2001). Questions throughout the chapter spark reflection about one's goals, mission, and legacy.

MICROPRACTICES

MICROPRACTICE: DETERMINE YOUR STRENGTHS, VALUES, AND CONTRIBUTIONS

There are many resources for reflecting on one's strengths, values, and contributions. Select from the following list to develop great self-awareness, legacy mapping, and professional strengths.

- To get to know your signature strengths for strength-based leadership:
  - Complete the strengths finders survey (Rath & Conchie, 2008): https://store.gallup.com/p/en-us/10369/strengths-based-leadership
- To see how your top values dovetail and support your leadership strengths:
  - Complete the VIA's Character Strengths Survey (Values Institute on Character, n.d.): https://www.viacharacter.org/survey/account/Register

- To guide you in reflecting on life's greatest questions, "What are you doing for others? What is your mission and purpose?"
  - Complete the contribify profile (Rath, 2020): https://contribify.com/book/lifes-great-question
- To read a more complete reflection for legacy leadership:
  - *Legacy leadership: The application workbook* (Sandstrom, J., 2017)

MICROPRACTICE: LEGACY MAPPING

Hinds et al. (2015) developed a systematic way to create a career legacy map with intention and purpose. Legacy mapping to plan for and document meaningful work in nursing begins with two questions (Hinds et al., 2015):

- What do you want to improve in nursing through your efforts?
- What would you like to be best known for?

MICROPRACTICE: SAGE LETTER

Write yourself a Sage Letter. Imagine that you are 70 years old looking back on your career. Write a letter to your younger self and explain the lessons you learned, the reputation you developed, and the legacy that you created during your working years. Or consider writing a letter to the future self you aspire to become. Explore this resource, http://www.futureme.org, for further guidance.

LEARNING NARRATIVE BY DAN PESUT

I had the opportunity to contribute a chapter to a book edited by William Rosa (2016), *Nurses as Leaders: Evolutionary Visions of Nursing Leadership*. The book is an excellent resource full of inspiration and stories of many nursing leaders and their contributions through time. Each chapter is a learning narrative. The title of my chapter was "Transformed and In Service: Creating the Future Through Renewal." In this chapter, I share my professional journey and path to becoming a nurse. I also share some legacy contributions related to my time as President of the Honor Society of Nursing, Sigma Theta Tau International (2003–2005). My presidential call to action was "Create the Future Through Renewal" (Pesut, 2004). I challenged Sigma members to consider the most meaningful activities that support personal and professional renewal. One of several outcomes I identified for the 2003–2005 biennium was the creation of a resource paper on reflective practice in nursing (Freshwater et al., 2005). The foreword I wrote to that report details my logic about the importance of reflective practice and personal and professional renewal. I also believe it crystallizes my leadership legacy intentions both at the time and today. I wrote:

> Personally, and professionally, I believe reflection is a means of renewal. My logic goes something like this: As self is renewed, commitments to service come forward more easily. Renewed commitments to service require attention to mindfulness and reflective

practice. Mindful reflective practice begets questions that support inquiry. Such inquiry guides knowledge work and evidence-based care giving. Care giving supports society as knowledge, values, and service intersect. Knowledgeable people and especially knowledgeable nurses provide care that society needs. Creating a caring society is the spirit work of nursing. Creating a caring society starts with nurses caring for themselves and becoming, through reflection, more conscious and intentional in their being, thinking, feeling, doing, and acting. Reflection is a form of "inner work" that results in the energy for engaging in "outer service." Reflection in-and-on action supports meaning-making and purpose management in one's professional life.

The nursing scholars who have participated in the development of this resource paper are to be commended. They have devoted many long hours to the creation of this document. They have role modeled for all of us the creation and development of a learning community dedicated to enhancing knowledge, learning, and service. They created a global transcendent team and have demonstrated the value and benefits of global cooperation around a very important professional developmental concept and practice for nurses. I admire and appreciate the work and effort this team has put forth and am pleased to introduce their work to the members of the honor society and nurses throughout the world.

I think there are many stimulating and provocative ideas in this resource paper. If reflective practice is new to you, I hope that the ideas and resources you discover will stimulate your curiosity and enable you to see your work in nursing through new ways. If reflective practice is already familiar to you, I hope that you support and encourage others to experiment with the notions, information, and resources gathered together in this paper. As we collectively reflect on the professional purpose of nursing, I am certain the spirit of nursing will be renewed. As members of the Honor Society of Nursing, Sigma Theta Tau International, each of us has a responsibility to enact the virtues of love, honor, and courage that are part of our heritage. As we develop our capacity and commitment for reflection, we will affirm that spirit of nursing and make nursing-care differences in the lives of people for whom we care. (Pesut, 2014, p. 1)

I invite readers to access the report (freely available in the Sigma Repository at https://sigma.nursingrepository.org/handle/10755/621207) and appreciate the legacy leadership it represents 18 years later. In fact, the people who worked on that task force have created a program of scholarship and their own legacies related to reflective practice in the nursing profession (Freshwater et al., 2009; Horton-Deutsch & Sherwood, 2017; Sherwood & Horton-Deutsch, 2015; Wei & Horton-Deutsch, 2022). The knowledge work and programs of scholarship about reflective practice initiated in 2005 continue today and are an example of leadership reimagined with a legacy perspective in mind.

Consider the following questions after you have studied the report:

1. What are applications of key resources in the white paper across education, practice, and research?

   _____

   _____

   _____

2. How does the report inform education and ways to better prepare nurses for contemporary practice?

   _____

   _____

   _____

3. What research questions remain to validate the evidence base for integrating reflective practice into nurses' work?

   _____

   _____

   _____

REFLECTIVE QUESTIONS

1. How do I enact the legacy leadership principles and practices in my work?

   _____

   _____

   _____

2. How do my strengths, values, and contributions influence my thinking about legacy leadership?

   _____

   _____

   _____

3. What lessons am I teaching in each interaction I have?

_____

_____

_____

4. What stories will people share about me in the future?

_____

_____

_____

5. What will others learn from those stories?

_____

_____

_____

6. What is more important to me, the results I achieve or how I achieve them?

_____

_____

_____

7. Have I made the impact I want in my work?

_____

_____

_____

8. What will colleagues remember about me as someone who made a difference in their lives?

_____

_____

_____

9. How have I put a system in place that enables people to feel connected and a sense of belonging, commitment, and dedication to their work accordingly?

_____

_____

_____

REFERENCES

Freshwater, D., Horton-Deutsch, S., Sherwood, G. D., & Taylor, B. J. (2005). *The scholarship of reflective practice.* https://sigma.nursingrepository.org/handle/10755/621207

Freshwater, D., Taylor, B., & Sherwood, G. (2009). International textbook of reflective practice in nursing. *Neonatal Network, 28*(3), 31–32.

Hinds, P. S., Britton, D. R., Coleman, L., Engh, E., Humbel, T. K., Keller, S., Kelly, K. P., Menard, J., Lee, M. A., Roberts-Turner, R., & Walczak, D. (2015). Creating a career legacy map to help assure meaningful work in nursing. *Nursing Outlook, 63*(2), 211–218. https://doi.org/10.1016/j.outlook.2014.08.002

Horton-Deutsch, S., & Sherwood, G. D. (2017). *Reflective practice: Transforming education and improving outcomes* (2nd ed.). Sigma Theta Tau International.

Kouzes, J., & Posner, B. (2006). *A leader's legacy.* Jossey-Bass. https://psycnet.apa.org/record/2006-10933-000

Pesut, D. J. (2004). Create the future through renewal. *Reflections on Nursing Leadership, 30*(1), 24–25, 56. https://archives.iupui.edu/bitstream/handle/2450/12067/Mss051_Presidential-Call-to-Action_2003-2005.pdf?sequence=1&isAllowed=y

Pesut, D. J. (2014). Foreword. In D. Freshwater, S. Horton-Deutsch, G. Sherwood, & B. Taylor, *The scholarship of reflective practice.* Sigma Theta Tau International. https://sigma.nursingrepository.org/bitstream/handle/10755/621207/Paper.pdf?sequence=1&isAllowed=y

Rath, T. (2020). *Life's great question: Discover how you contribute to the world.* Tom Rath.

Rath, T., & Conchie, B. (2008). *Strengths based leadership.* Gallup Press.

Rosa, W. (2016). *Nurses as leaders: Evolutionary visions of nursing leadership.* Springer.

Sandstrom, J. (2017). *Legacy leadership: The application workbook.* Coachworks Press.

Sandstrom, J., & Smith, L. (2001). *Legacy leadership: The 5 best practices at-a-glance.* https://coachworks.com/legacyleadership/pdfs/LL_At-A-Glance_0508.pdf

Sandstrom, J., & Smith, L. (2017). *Legacy leadership: The leader's guide to lasting greatness* (2nd ed.). Coachworks Press.

Sherwood, G., & Horton-Deutsch, S. (2015). *Reflective organizations: On the front lines of QSEN & reflective practice implementation.* Sigma Theta Tau International.

VIA Institute on Character. (n.d.). *About the VIA Institute on Character.* https://www.viacharacter.org/about

Wei, H., & Horton-Deutsch, S. (2022). *Visionary leadership in healthcare.* Sigma Theta Tau International.

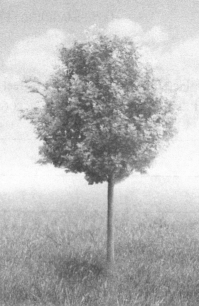

CHAPTER 15

REFLECTIVE PRACTICE, UNITARY CARING SCIENCE, AND WISDOM: THE HEART OF THE CAPACITY TO GROW

Sara Horton-Deutsch, PhD, RN, ANEF, SGAHN, FAAN
Gisela van Rensburg, DLitt et Phil, RN, RM, RPN, RCN, RNE, RNA, ROrthN, FANSA

LEARNING OBJECTIVES

- Describe reflective practice and Caring Science's underlying ethical, moral, and philosophical worldviews.

- Appreciate the essential nature of reflection for personal and professional growth.

- Value individual and relational practices in reflection.

- Explore ways to connect more deeply and wisely with others.

- Unite personal, relational (professional), and organizational ways of understanding our way of being, doing, and becoming in the world.

BEFORE YOU BEGIN

This final chapter explores healing and caring from a spiritual and philosophical perspective. It emphasizes the importance of heart-centered consciousness in interactions with others. It provides guidelines on how to achieve this, such as pausing and slowing down, standing by our core values, unlocking our fears, and speaking our truth from the heart. When preparing to facilitate learners in micropractices, learners benefit when educators share their experiences, modeling the way for others. Like other micropractices throughout this textbook, the micropractice may be reflected upon, journaled, shared, discussed, or combined. Opportunities for dialogue allow educators to assess and evaluate learning and provide affirmation and confirmation of learner experiences.

This chapter focuses on individual and relational ways of working from the heart. As an individual practice, the courageous caring moment concept encourages readers to reflect on a time when they could rise above challenges and display courage. Educators are encouraged to share moments of courage in their careers and then have students reflect and journal on one of their own. Next, the chapter introduces the Seven Sacred Sutras (Watson, 2021), which are contemplative meditations to connect to one's source, soul, and the sacred. The sutras shared are stillness, silence, solitude, spirit, simplicity, service, and surrender. Learners may be encouraged to practice these sutras and explore their own preparatory practices for remaining heart-centered.

Beyond individual practices, the chapter explores ways to work more heart-centered with others. It discusses the concept of healing/Caritas circles, which are welcoming environments that create a warm atmosphere for open-hearted, deeply human, and caring interactions. These circles involve guided visualization, music, reading, meditation, silence, and poetry. The text also suggests that individuals can hold a circle for themselves, a Circle of One, to listen to their inner voices and follow their intuition. Educators are encouraged to explore the application of healing/Caritas circles for creating healthy and healing work environments. Another teaching moment is considering how the circle framework can be modified and used in clinical and academic settings.

The chapter introduces the 5-D cycle of appreciative inquiry as another relational practice. This method can reflect on successes and strengths, identify what works well, and find ways to build on it. The 5-D cycle is applied through the lens of Unitary Caring Science and is guided by the 10 Caritas Processes. Educators can have learners work in small groups to practice the 5-D cycle as applied to their work settings or be provided a workplace scenario to work from.

KEY CHAPTER THEMES:

1. *Heart-centered consciousness and caring*

2. *Courageous caring moments*

3. *Seven Sacred Sutras*

4. *Healing/Caritas circles*

5. *5-D cycle of appreciative inquiry and 10 Caritas Processes*

Chapter 15 guides expanded personal growth and spiritual development, focusing on healing, caring, and self-reflection. It provides micropractices and exercises for individuals and groups, promoting a deeper understanding of oneself and interactions with others. It benefits learners to expand their personal development, spirituality, and holistic healing practices. It provides practical tools and strategies that can be applied in various contexts, from personal, professional, and leadership development, in alignment with the AACN Essentials (2019).

MICROPRACTICES

COURAGEOUS CARING MOMENT

Think of a time when you experienced a courageous caring moment, a time you were able to rise above the hurt, disappointment, conflict, and uncertainty.

QUESTIONS FOR REFLECTION

1. Where did your courage come from?

_____

_____

2. What core value(s) was present?

_____

_____

3. Now think about the story/situation …

    a. What did you feel?

        _____

        _____

    b. What did you see?

        _____

        _____

    c. What did you do?

        _____

        _____

    d. What did you say?

        _____

        _____

    e. How did you love?

        _____

        _____

QUESTIONS FOR DEEPER REFLECTION

1. Why do you think this moment continues to stand out to you now?

_____

_____

2. What difference did this make then?

_____

_____

3. What difference has it made through time for you, your organization, family, community, and the world?

_____

_____

JEAN WATSON'S SEVEN SACRED SUTRAS

Sacred sutras are words or phrases that are studied, recited, and contemplated upon as a means of deepening one's understanding of spiritual truths and achieving spiritual growth. They help us to claim what we stand for and value, guiding us along our spiritual journey. They are considered repositories of wisdom, enlightenment, and liberation. Review the following sutras:

1. Stillness

2. Silence

3. Solitude

4. Spirit

5. Simplicity

6. Service

7. Surrender

Now, contemplate your sutras and write your responses below.

1. What words guide you to your truth?

_____

_____

2. How might the practice of your sutras help you to be more present, develop insight and wisdom, and find peace and contentment?

_____

_____

NOBLE VIRTUES

The following noble virtues are sets of moral and situational guidelines within which one functions:

1. *Right view:* This refers to the respect that we show our patients, the community, and our colleagues. When assessing a patient, it should be done objectively and without any prejudice.

2. *Right thought:* Ensure all information, actions, or incidents are reported diligently and correctly. Do a comprehensive assessment and do not rush. Respect the human dignity of all your patients, their loved ones, and your colleagues.

3. *Right speech:* Always act professionally and as a role model when addressing patients, community members, or colleagues. Choose your words carefully and make sure the person understands you. It often is not what you say but how you say it.

4. *Right action:* Ensure that your conduct is always professional. This requires competent nurses who are committed to continuous professional development. The fact that you have completed your course does not mean that you are going to stop improving your competence or learning new skills.

5. *Right living:* This refers to one's actions, thoughts, and speech. Engage in actions that do not cause any harm, physically or psychologically; always be honest (e.g., when reporting on the condition of a patient). Ensure that all actions are meaningful.

6. *Right effort:* Our professional conduct must be of such a nature that we are seen as leaders in the professional community. We must ask ourselves how much effort we are putting into what we are doing and how we are doing it. The right effort will require deliberate self-development.

7. *Right mindfulness:* In realizing this we should be mindful of what we are thinking, saying, and doing. Have a positive attitude and treat everyone with respect.

8. *Right concentration:* The last element refers to the cognitive processes. Through reflection-on-action and reflection-in-action, the right knowledge will be developed.

Various models exist with different virtues. Caring for the self and others, guided by the eight ancient principles, can steer us when reflecting on our positions as nurses and change agents. Review the noble truths above and contemplate how they resonate with you.

Are there others you would add?

_____

_____

LEARNING NARRATIVE

Using the 5-D cycle of appreciative inquiry (Hammond, 2013), the 10 Caritas Processes (Watson, 2021), and emergent strategies as a guide, plan to deliver a healing or wisdom circle. Here are some individual and group reflection questions to get started.

INDIVIDUAL REFLECTION:

1. Why are you calling a circle?

_____

_____

2. Where does hosting this circle fit into your life?

_____

_____

3. How does it serve your soul/your own wholeness?

_____

_____

4. Whom would you enjoy co-hosting the circle with?

_____

_____

GROUP REFLECTION:

1. Share your ideas of what makes an effectively functioning relationship between co-hosts.

_____

_____

2. How can you support each other?

_____

_____

3. What is the intention of the circle?

_____

_____

4. Whom would you like to welcome into the circle, and how will you invite and reach out to them (if known/if unknown)?

_____

_____

5. Where will you host the circle?

_____

_____

6. How would you like to prepare the physical space to ensure circle members will feel welcome and safe?

_____

_____

REFLECTIVE QUESTIONS

1. How does my understanding and appreciation for the value of experiential knowledge expand in an environment that promotes reflective practices?

_____

_____

_____

2. In what ways do I already practice reflectively? How can I deepen practice through the lens of Unitary Caring Science?

_____

_____

_____

3. How do reflective practice and Unitary Caring Science guide me to embodied wisdom?

_____

_____

_____

4. What are the needs of educational and practice settings to promote reflection and Unitary Caring Science in teaching, learning, and service?

_____

_____

_____

5. How am I continually nurturing and cultivating my ways of being and becoming more human? How congruent are my practices with the principles of Unitary Caring Science?

_____

_____

_____

6. How can I use individual, relational, and group/organizational reflective practices to expand caring consciousness and embodied wisdom?

_____

_____

_____

REFERENCES

American Association of Colleges of Nursing. (2021). *The essentials: Core competencies for professional nursing education.* https://www.aacnnursing.org/Portals/42/AcademicNursing/pdf/Essentials-2021.pdf

Hammond, S. (2013). *The thin book of appreciative inquiry* (3rd ed.). Thin Book Publishing Co.

Watson, J. (2021). *Caring Science as sacred science.* (Rev. ed.). Lotus Library.